KU-196-780

Setting Your Weight

A Complete Programme

Fitness, Health & Nutrition was created by Rebus, Inc. and published by Time-Life Books.

REBUS, INC.

Publisher: RODNEY FRIEDMAN
Editorial Director: CHARLES L. MEE JR.

Editor: THOMAS DICKEY
Executive Editor: SUSAN BRONSON
Senior Editor: CARL LOWE
Associate Editors: MARY CROWLEY, WILLIAM DUNNETT
Contributing Editor: JACQUELINE DAMIAN
Copy Editor: LINDA EPSTEIN

Art Director: JUDITH HENRY
Designer: FRANCINE KASS
Photographer: STEVEN MAYS
Photo Stylist: NOLA LOPEZ
Photo Assistant: TIMOTHY JEFFS

Test Kitchen Director: GRACE YOUNG
Recipe Editor: BONNIE J. SLOTNICK
Contributing Editor: MARYA DALRYMPLE
Chief of Research: CARNEY W. MIMMS III
Assistant Editor: PENELOPE CLARK

TIME-LIFE BOOKS

European Executive Editor: Gillian Moore
Design Director: Ed Skyner
Assistant Design Director: Mary Staples
Chief of Research: Vanessa Kramer
Chief Sub-Editor: Ilse Gray

EUROPEAN EDITION

Designer: Sandra Doble
Sub-Editor: Lindsay McTeague
Chief of Editorial Production: Maureen Kelly
Production Assistant: Samantha Hill
Editorial Department: Theresa John, Debra Lelliott

FITNESS, HEALTH & NUTRITION

Setting Your Weight

A Complete Programme

Time-Life Books, Amsterdam

CONSULTANTS FOR THIS BOOK

Theodore B. Van Itallie, M.D., Professor of Medicine at the College of Physicians and Surgeons, Columbia University, is co-director of the Obesity Research Center at St. Luke's-Roosevelt Hospital Center/Rockefeller University, New York City.

Ann Grandjean, Ed. D., is chief nutrition consultant to the U.S. Olympic Committee and an instructor in the Sports Medicine Program, University of Nebraska Medical Center.

John White, Ph.D., is Reader in Human Sciences at the West London Institute of Higher Education, with responsibilities for undergraduate teaching and postgraduate research in exercise physiology.

Myron Winick, M.D., is Professor of Nutrition at Columbia University College of Physicians and Surgeons, New York.

Moya de Wet, a consultant nutritionist and State Registered Dietitian, took her degree in nutrition at the Polytechnic of North London.

Colonel Frederick R. Drews, who designed the exercise routines on pages 48-49 and 80-81, is a Doctor of Physical Education.

ISBN 0 7054 0717 9

TIME-LIFE is a trademark of Time Incorporated U.S.A.

This book is not intended as a medical guide or a substitute for the advice of a doctor. Readers, especially those who have or suspect they may have medical problems, especially those involving their weight, should consult a doctor about any suggestions made in this book. Readers beginning a programme of strenuous physical exercise are also urged to consult a doctor.

CONTENTS

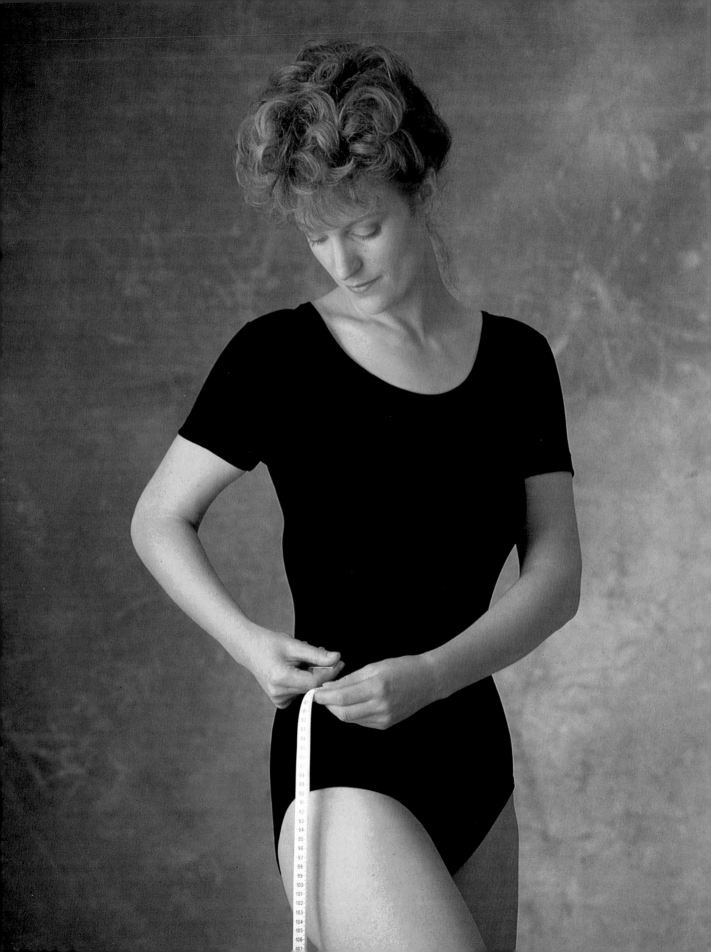

CHAPTER ONE

The Essentials of Weight Control

Why excess fat accumulates — and the right plan for taking it off

To lose weight safely and permanently, you need to alter both your eating habits and your exercise habits. Weight-loss programmes that stress only what you eat and that place you on special diets that differ radically from what you normally eat do not produce long-term weight loss.

That is why this is not a diet book — at least not in the sense that it provides a regimen for a rapid weight loss that you follow for a limited time only. Researchers studying subjects who have tried special diets — other than those administered in hospital settings — have found that such programmes seldom result in a permanent reduction in weight. As a rule, these diets may allow you to slim down, but once you resume your previous eating habits, your lost weight will return, often accompanied by extra kilograms you did not have before. To avoid this difficulty, you must change your daily routines, particularly what you eat and how active you are, and adopt practices that you can adhere to for the rest of your life.

Energy Balance: The Key to Gain and Loss

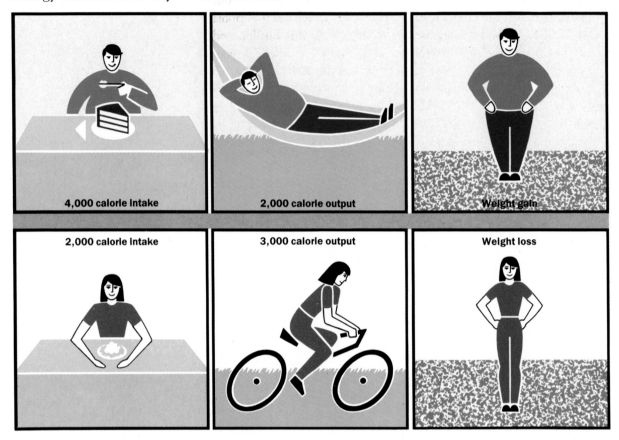

4,000 calorie intake

2,000 calorie output

Weight gain

2,000 calorie intake

3,000 calorie output

Weight loss

When your energy intake (supplied by food) is in balance with your energy output (expended to sustain daily activities), your weight stays relatively stable. However, when intake is greater than output — as measured in calories — the excess calories are stored as body fat and you will gain weight *(top)*. To lose weight, you need to tip this energy balance by consuming fewer calories and increasing your physical activity until output exceeds intake. Your body will then turn to the stored fat for energy, causing weight loss *(bottom)*.

What causes you to become overweight?

The energy contained in the food you consume — which your body absorbs and uses to maintain its internal functions and power its day-to-day activities, including exercise — is the most important variable affecting your weight. When you eat foods that contain more energy than necessary to fuel your body and repair its structure, the metabolic processing of the excess nutrients results in the creation of body fat. The nutrients enter your bloodstream through the walls of your stomach or intestines, and instead of taking part in the chemical reactions that produce energy, these substances — whether they were originally dietary protein, carbohydrate or fat — are used to synthesize triglycerides, which are stored as body fat.

So the formula that produces significant weight loss and long-term maintenance of a desirable lower weight is a decrease in the amount of food energy you eat accompanied by an increase in the energy that your activities utilize. These changes in energy balance deprive your body of excess food energy it might store as fat and force it to draw on some of the energy stored in the fat that has already been accumulated.

Why should you control your weight?

Body fat, contained in adipose tissue, puts increased stress on your ligaments, tendons, bones and lean muscle tissue, which has to support the fat's weight. Keeping your weight down avoids this burden and makes it easier for you to move about during normal activities as well as during workouts. And being reasonably slender can benefit your back. Excess fat is often carried at the front of the abdomen, which can create a forward tug on the backbone. Losing that fat and keeping it off reduces this stressful pull.

While the exact physiological mechanisms that endow slim people with better health are not well understood, statistical studies of population groups have established that weighing less better enables you to undergo surgery without medical complications and, if you are a woman, to give birth more safely. Data compiled by life insurance companies in the United States show that men who are obese (20 per cent heavier than the statistical average) have a 20 per cent shorter life expectancy than the norm. Obese women have a 10 per cent shorter life expectancy than average women.

Many long-term studies have also shown that high-fat diets and excess weight are significant risk factors for a whole spectrum of life-threatening diseases, including hypertension, stroke, diabetes, gall bladder problems and certain types of cancer. The intake of dietary fat, particularly saturated fat, is associated with an elevated blood cholesterol level, a major factor in coronary heart disease.

For the overweight person, thick layers of insulating fat increase discomfort in hot weather. Normally, a significant amount of heat escapes from the body as the blood circulates through tissues just under the skin. But extra layers of fat tissue under the skin block this dissipation of heat. And, because overweight people radiate less heat than thin people do, they perspire more heavily to give off body heat through the evaporation of moisture from their skin.

According to today's standards of physical beauty, it is better to be slim than heavy, and there is a strong social stigma attached to being fat. Many people regard the overweight as weak-willed. Studies done by social scientists have found that heavier people may have more trouble getting a job than thinner people, their social interactions may be less satisfactory and their self-image and self-respect may suffer. Losing weight can sometimes alleviate these problems and make an important difference to how you see yourself and how others see you.

How do calories affect your weight?

The amount of energy contained in your food and the amount of energy used by your body are commonly expressed in calories. One calorie equals the amount of energy necessary to raise one gram of water one degree Celsius. Only carbohydrates, fats, proteins and alcohol contain calories. Water, fibre, vitamins and minerals do not contain any. (Because of variations in storage facilities, handling methods

and the conditions in which a food item was grown or raised, calorie counts for the same item may differ from one reading to the next.)

The amount of energy necessary to form half a kilogram of adipose tissue is approximately 3,500 calories. Therefore, to lose half a kilogram of fat-containing tissue, you have to burn up 3,500 more calories than you consume in your food.

Can't you just consume fewer calories in order to lose weight?

Trying to lose kilograms by eating less can cause weight loss. However, this strategy is not as effective for long-term weight reduction and maintenance of a lower weight as is a programme that combines exercise with a calorie-restricted diet.

Studies show that when you reduce dietary calories, your body may lower its resting metabolic rate, managing to get by on fewer calories. After a short period of dieting, to continue to lose weight you will have to restrict your food intake even more than you did at the beginning of your diet. And if you are eating a very limited amount of food, you are more likely to stop dieting. However, research on athletes and the overweight shows that exercising burns up more calories and allows you to eat more food while maintaining a caloric deficit between the amount you eat and the amount you use in daily activity.

Another problem you may confront if you try to lose weight solely by means of calorie restriction is that your body will not merely use its own fat for energy; it will also utilize a significant amount of muscle tissue to supply its energy needs. This is undesirable since it is your excess fat, not your lean tissue, that is related to problems such as hypertension and diabetes (although researchers have not isolated the mechanisms by which it contributes to these conditions). Studies of dieters show that those who work out lose less muscle tissue and a higher percentage of fat than those who are inactive.

What kind of exercise is the best for losing weight?

Any regular exercise routine that you find convenient is probably suitable. However, to burn the most calories per minute, you have to perform an aerobic exercise — such as running, cycling or brisk walking — that involves the repeated motion of the large muscle groups in the arms or legs. These endurance activities can be sustained for relatively long periods and so can burn up more calories than anaerobic exercises, such as weight lifting or sprinting, which are performed more intensely but for much shorter periods. Moreover, researchers have found that an aerobic exercise performed for at least 20 minutes draws on fat for at least 50 per cent of its energy. Conversely, anaerobic activities draw more heavily on glycogen, the starch stored in the muscles and liver, to fuel their motion.

Won't exercising make you hungrier and liable to eat more?

Contrary to what you might expect, studies show that an intense ex-

ercise session tends to decrease your appetite and cause you to eat less at your next meal than you normally would. And, while it is true that if you exercise consistently you may increase your total food intake, your energy output may more than compensate. A study of middle-aged joggers found that even though they consistently consumed more calories daily than their sedentary counterparts, they weighed less than the men and women in the study who did not exercise.

Does shedding excess fat reverse the health hazards of being overweight?

Losing weight does mitigate the health risks associated with being overweight; moreover, studies have established that you do not have to lose a large amount of weight to improve your health. For instance, a loss of as little as 3 kilograms can significantly lower the blood-sugar level of some diabetics. And similarly small weight losses have been shown to lower both elevated blood cholesterol levels and blood pressure, important indicators of cardiovascular health.

Is all fat unhealthy?

No. In fact, you cannot live without some fat. Carbohydrates and fat are your main sources of energy for the metabolic processes that keep you alive and enable you to move about. But by weight, fat is the most energy-dense source of fuel; it supplies twice as much energy per kilogram as carbohydrates. This is possible because most of your fat consists of triglycerides, chemicals whose molecular construction makes them efficient energy-storage centres. The digestive and metabolic processes convert dietary fat to body fat.

When you perform a low-intensity exercise such as slow jogging, your body gets about half of its energy from its carbohydrate reserves and about half from its reserves of fat (as well as a small amount from protein). But when you run or exercise for two hours or more, you exhaust most of your carbohydrate reserves. Your body must then rely mainly on its fat reserves to provide muscular energy.

In addition to its role as fuel for movement and exercise, essential fat, which is located in your muscle tissue, heart, lungs, liver and other organs, takes part in these organs' necessary physiological functions by absorbing, storing and transporting the fat-soluble vitamins (A, D, E and K). These vitamins, dissolved in essential fat, are catalysts for vital metabolic functions such as the creation of blood-clotting factors in the liver. Ingested fat also supplies essential fatty acids and helps delay the emptying of the stomach so that digestion can take place. Finally, essential fat forms the outer protective covering of nerves and is needed in cell membranes.

Women normally have a larger proportion of essential fat than men because they have fat deposited in the breasts, upper thighs, hips and buttocks. This extra fat is necessary for reproduction and provides energy used in the production of milk for nursing.

How Fat Forms

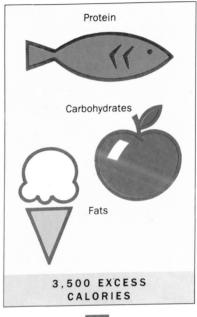

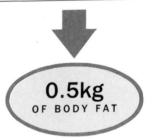

Body fat forms not only from dietary fat, but from protein and carbohydrates as well. Though dietary fat contains more calories per gram than the other two nutrients, any food supplying calories that are not burnt up in daily activity will be converted into fat. An excess of 3,500 calories — whether consumed over a week or a year — will increase body fat by approximately half a kilogram.

What Happens to Fat Cells

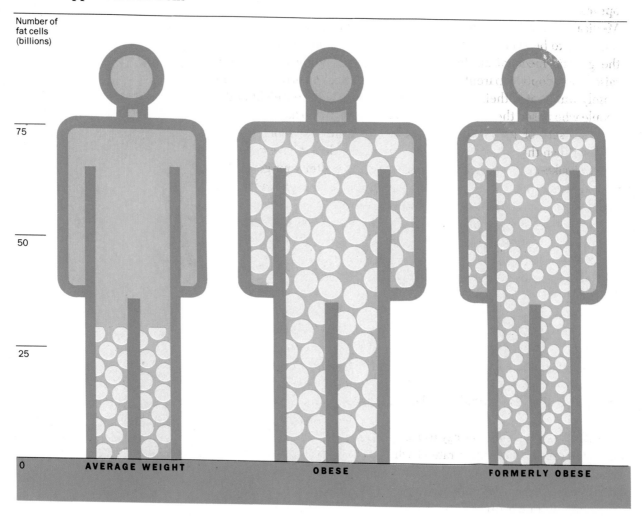

Number of
fat cells
(billions)

75

50

25

0

AVERAGE WEIGHT   OBESE   FORMERLY OBESE

A person of average weight has one third as many fat cells as an obese person *(left and centre)* — 25 to 30 billion fat cells as compared with 75 billion. The average amount of fat within each fat cell is about 35 per cent greater in the obese. Any weight loss occurs solely through a decrease in cell size *(right)*, and when the obese lose weight, their fat cells can shrink to about one third the size of cells in non-obese people. The number of fat cells remains the same, however; the cells will expand again if the lost weight is regained.

What happens to your body when you lose weight?

Researchers studying fat cells believe that while most of those cells are created early in life, overeating as an adult may produce additional fat cells. When you lose weight, the fat cells will shrink as the body draws on their triglyceride content to meet its energy needs. But these fat cells will never vanish entirely; indeed, they will actually fill up with triglycerides again if you consume too many calories, causing you to regain the weight you lost.

Some researchers have theorized that this physiological process occurs because of a human evolutionary adaptation. In epochs when famines occurred frequently, human survival may have depended on the body's use of the fat that had been stored when a surplus of food was available. Now that surplus food is generally available all the time in the developed countries of the world, the body's mechanism for storing this fat in adipose tissue has become an impediment to weight loss and a threat to health.

12

If your parents are fat, will you have to struggle to maintain your optimal weight?

Medical researchers believe that some people have an inherited tendency to be overweight, although scientists do not yet understand the genetic mechanisms by which this occurs. Studies of children raised by adoptive parents show that their weight correlates more closely with that of their biological parents than with the weight of the people who raised them. Studies of identical twins, who have inherited identical sets of genes, show that their weights are more closely matched than the weights of fraternal twins, who do not have the same genetic make-up. Nevertheless, while you cannot alter your genes, almost all weight-control researchers agree that your lifestyle and eating habits are significant, controllable factors that affect your weight.

Your eating habits — how much you eat, when you eat and what kinds of foods you eat — form a behaviour pattern that you originally learnt from your parents and your peers. Habits such as always eating everything on your plate or ending your meal with a rich dessert are acquired behaviour traits that can contribute to being overweight. Replacing these habits with others is called behaviour modification. Many researchers believe that behaviour modification holds the key to weight control for most overweight people, particularly those who have dieted repeatedly but failed to achieve permanent weight loss. With their own efforts and sometimes with professional help, many people can learn new attitudes and behaviour patterns.

How do you gauge your energy usage?

Scientists call the minimum rate at which your body uses energy the basal metabolic rate. Your body is at this basal rate first thing in the morning, before you get started with your daily activities. This rate is the minimum rate of energy use that the body needs to carry out critical functions while at rest. These functions include maintaining body temperature, breathing, circulation, cellular metabolism and glandular activity. The basal metabolic rate for adults varies from 0.8 to 1.4 calories per minute, according to weight, sex, body composition (amount of muscle tissue) and other factors. Your resting metabolic rate, your rate of energy usage when you are relaxing during the day, is only slightly higher than your basal rate.

The highest rate of energy output is called the thermic effect of exercise, or thermogenesis, the scientific term for your increased energy usage when you are actively using your muscles. A 68-kilogram man whose metabolism uses one calorie per minute during sleep may expend 12 calories a minute during intense exercise such as running or swimming. Some researchers also believe that your metabolism remains elevated for several hours after you finish exercising, but this has not been definitely established.

There is another thermic effect, called the thermic effect of food. This term refers to the increased rate of energy usage that takes place for several hours after a meal as your body expends energy to digest your food and move it through the alimentary canal.

If you seem to gain weight easily, is it because your metabolism is sluggish?

If you have a low resting metabolic rate, it is not because your metabolism is inherently sluggish; it is a matter of having a low level of muscle mass. A low resting metabolic rate can cause you to gain weight more easily and have a harder time losing it than someone whose metabolic rate is relatively high. A person with more muscle and a high metabolic rate uses up more energy per minute and is less prone to store food energy as fat than someone with a lower rate. This means that the person with a so-called fast metabolism burns more calories when doing the same activity — even watching television.

The variability of your body's energy usage reduces the usefulness of a restricted diet as your sole means of losing weight. When you consume fewer calories than normal, your body cuts down its energy use in an effort to conserve the energy it takes from your diet, and your metabolic rate decreases. Precisely how it accomplishes this is not clear. But just as the mechanism for storing fat in adipose tissue may have originated as an adaptation to famine, your body's energy-conserving reaction to a restricted diet may be an evolutionary response designed to ensure survival during periods of food scarcity.

Do you inevitably gain weight as you get older?

Although most people tend to gain weight as they get older, it has not been determined how much of this weight gain is due to decreased physical activity and how much is due to the physiological aspects of ageing. Studies have shown that older people generally use up energy at a slower rate than younger people: basal metabolism drops by approximately 4 per cent per decade throughout adulthood. This lowered metabolic rate might make more food energy available for creating adipose tissue as you age, even though your calorie intake is the same.

Are there surgical techniques that can help you lose weight quickly?

For most people, the risks involved in surgery designed to help them lose weight far outweigh the benefits. These drastic measures are suited only to those for whom obesity is life-threatening.

One operation that is designed to bring about weight loss is gastric reduction surgery, or gastroplasty, a procedure that shrinks the stomach by stapling part of it closed or that fills up part of the stomach with an inflated balloon. After this procedure, it should take less food to make you feel full; overeating will cause nausea. When your appetite and food intake diminish, of course, you will probably lose weight. However, eventually your stomach will stretch, allowing you to eat as much as you did before the operation. A disadvantage of this

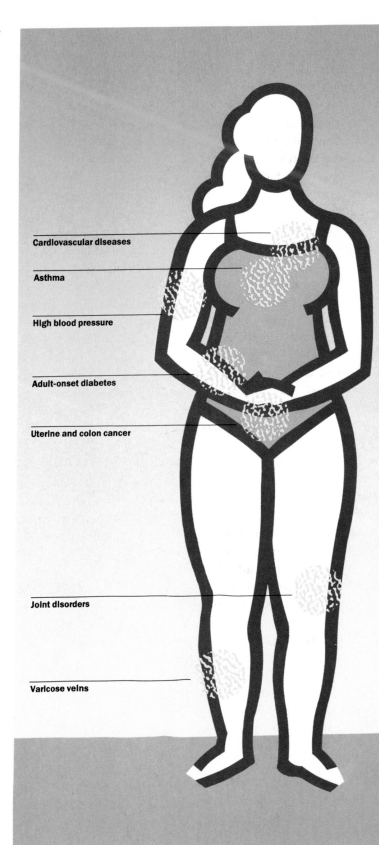

Cardiovascular diseases

Asthma

High blood pressure

Adult-onset diabetes

Uterine and colon cancer

Joint disorders

Varicose veins

Health Risks of Obesity

Doctors have observed for years that obesity is associated with ill health, and clinical evidence for this has been accumulating. The risk of the conditions indicated on the left rises significantly when a person exceeds his or her desirable weight by 20 per cent.

The most common physical ailment of the obese is hypertension. People who are 45 and older are twice as likely to have high blood pressure as their thinner contemporaries; in people younger than 45, the risk is almost six times greater. Many studies have also linked excess body fat with elevated blood cholesterol and increased incidence of heart attack and stroke. Some experts think that the risk of heart disease increases by 30 per cent in people who are 20 to 30 per cent overweight, and by 100 per cent for those who are more than 40 per cent overweight. Diabetes is three times more prevalent among the obese, and research has determined that overweight people are at above average risk from uterine and colon cancer.

The obese are also at greater risk from conditions such as asthma, bronchitis, varicose veins, and joint and muscle complaints.

With weight loss, virtually all of these health problems can be reduced or eliminated. For example, in an Australian study, hypertensives who lost an average of 8 kilograms saw their blood pressure drop significantly. Among diabetics, losing even a small amount of weight may lower blood sugar levels. And a major study indicated that each 10 per cent reduction in weight in men 35 to 55 years old would result in about a 20 per cent decrease in the incidence of coronary heart disease.

15

method is that it does not re-educate a person to change his or her eating habits. Moreover, some people who have this type of surgery suffer spleen injury and other complications.

Plastic surgery to suck the fat out from under your skin — suction lipectomy — cannot remove enough fat to benefit the very over-weight. In addition, its effects cannot be guaranteed. Studies show that if eating patterns and lifestyle that caused the build-up of fat continue after the operation, fat that was removed by this procedure will return.

What is a realistic rate of weight loss?

A realistic goal is to lose between 0.5 and 1 kilogram per week. Studies show that people who have taken weight off and kept it off usually lose an average of half a kilogram per week. Gradual weight reduction is more successful than rapid weight loss because it requires only slight changes in behaviour that are easier to stick to for a long period of time than are radical changes. In addition, you are more likely to lose fat than muscle when your weight loss is gradual.

Since each half-kilogram of adipose tissue represents 3,500 calories, losing half a kilogram a week requires that you burn up one seventh of that amount per day, or at least 500 calories more than you eat. Your calorie deficit should be created by a combination of calorie-burning physical activity and dietary restriction.

Is there a limit to how much weight you can lose?

The set-point theory of weight maintenance contends that for any given level of physical activity, your body has a pre-set weight and body-fat percentage that it strives to maintain, no matter how much or how little food you eat. Set-point theorists believe that a part of your brain called the hypothalamus orchestrates your metabolism and other internal processes in an effort to stay at this steady set point by varying the rate at which you burn calories.

According to the set-point theory, if your level of physical activity remains constant, merely dieting to lose weight is extremely difficult since your body will automatically slow down its metabolic usage of calories to compensate for the reduced supply.

To support the set-point theory, proponents point to the fact that even though Americans consume 10 per cent fewer calories than they did 15 years ago, their average weight during that time has increased by about 2.5 kilograms. What has raised Americans' weight, they claim, is a decrease in activity, not an increase in food, and they hold that obesity is a disease of the sedentary, not of the gluttonous. They believe that exercise is the *only* viable way to control your weight.

However, the advocates of this theory have not been able to identify a specific physiological mechanism by which the hypothalamus or any other part of the body can keep your weight at a particular level. And their theory does not account for the fact that although it is difficult to lose weight by diet alone, it is still possible.

Lose Fat, Not Muscle

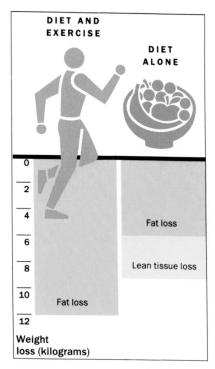

DIET AND EXERCISE

DIET ALONE

0
2
4
6 — Fat loss
8 — Lean tissue loss
10 — Fat loss
12

Weight loss (kilograms)

Combining diet with exercise not only helps promote a more effective loss of body fat, but helps ensure that you lose fat, not muscle mass. In one study, a group that simply reduced food intake lost an average of 9 kilograms in two months, while a group that added exercise to their programme lost 12 kilograms. Furthermore, as the chart above shows, 36 per cent of the weight lost in the diet-only group was muscle mass; in the diet-and-exercise group, all the weight lost was fat.

What causes weight-loss plateaus?
Why some dieters reach so-called plateaus, when their weight loss comes to a temporary halt, has not been fully explained, although many weight plateaus may be due to water retention. These plateaus are so common that many researchers in the field consider them to be a normal part of most weight-loss programmes. One way to get past a plateau is to increase your weekly exercise and cut back even further on your dietary calories until you begin to lose weight again.

Is it harder for women to lose weight than it is for men?
The fact that many societies expect women to be thinner than men, and that women therefore diet more often to lose weight, may have created the misconception that it is harder for women to lose weight than it is for men. But there are no scientific data to support that notion. Assuming a man and a woman each want to lose the same amount of body fat, neither one has an inborn advantage over the other in his or her effort to do so.

The same equality, however, does not hold true for weight maintenance. Because women's bodies normally contain a higher percentage of fat and a lower percentage of lean body mass than men's do, in order to maintain a constant, comparable weight, a woman needs to consume fewer calories than a man does. Since the male body consists of a larger proportion of muscle and therefore has a higher metabolic rate than a comparable female body, men may be able to eat more than women without adding adipose tissue.

What is the best way to get rid of cellulite?
Cellulite is a term that was popularized in European spas in the early 20th century to describe unsightly bumps and ripples of fat on the thighs and buttocks. The term was revived in the 1970s, and recent proponents of a cellulite theory argue that this is a special kind of fat, containing water, connective tissue and some waste products that normal fat lacks. Supposedly, women have more of a problem than men do with cellulite because of their hormonal balance, and also because the way in which fat lies beneath the skin differs between the sexes.

However, microscopic comparisons of normal fat tissue with lumpy "cellulite" fat tissue have not established any real difference between the two: their chemical composition is identical. Lumpy-looking fat occurs when cells containing fat increase in size and bulge out of the connective fibre compartments that usually contain them, giving skin a cross-hatched waffled appearance. But except for differences in appearance, all fat stored in the body's adipose tissue is identical.

Can you control where the fat comes off when you lose weight?
The way fat is distributed on your body and the places it comes off when you lose weight are both genetically determined. It is impossible to spot-reduce by exercising a particular body part or set of muscles.

How Fat Comes Off

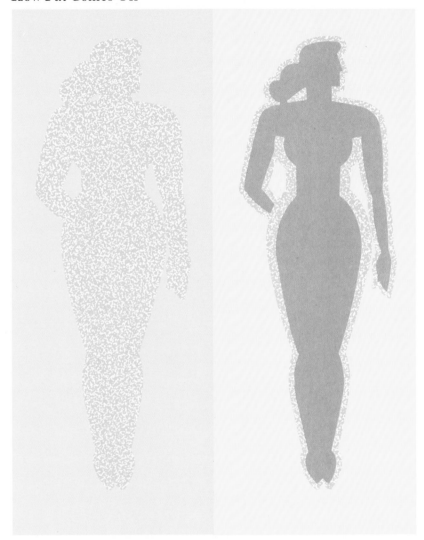

How does body shape change during a weight-loss programme? Researchers studied 42 overweight women on a diet-and-exercise regimen. They found that, at each 2.5 kilogram weight-loss interval, the amount of fat tissue lost in the trunk region was twice that lost in the arms and legs, as shown on the right. The study also revealed that fat was lost more quickly in the lower body, particularly the abdomen, hips and buttocks, than in the upper body. Even the wrists and ankles showed reduced measurements after a weight loss of about 10 kilograms.

When you lose weight, the fat deposits that are depleted as your body fat decreases are not affected by the type of exercise you perform. Doing exercises such as sit-ups for your stomach will strengthen your stomach muscles, but they will not, by themselves, cause fat to disappear from your abdominal area. Eventually, as you follow an exercise and diet programme, this and all your adipose tissue will shrink, but spot-reducing exercises, unless they contribute to an overall calorie deficit, will not speed this loss.

How does your body shape change as you lose weight?

Your body measurements do not change proportionally to the amount of weight you lose. Research on women who were dieting showed that the more kilograms these women lost, the more their measurements decreased. On average, the second 2.5 kilograms they lost reduced their measurements by twice as much as the first 2.5 kilograms did.

Body change during weight loss, therefore, is not a steady, constant process. If you are losing weight and do not immediately see a dramatic difference in your appearance, you should not let this fact demoralize you. Additional weight loss will probably make up for this apparent initial lack of progress.

Will eating particular foods and avoiding others help you lose weight faster?

Basically, the amount of weight you lose or gain comes down to a balance between the number of calories that you eat and the number that you expend. If you consume too much of any kind of food, no matter what its composition or nutritional content, the calories that it contains can contribute to your weight gain.

However, protein and carbohydrates are not quite as easily converted into storage fat as are fatty foods — another reason your diet should be low in fat. Furthermore, such complex carbohydrates as the starches contained in rice, whole-grain products, beans, peas and some vegetables are particularly recommended to dieters because they usually contain a substantial amount of fibre, the indigestible part of plants that has no usable calories because it passes right through the body without being absorbed.

Can you lose weight quickly on a high-protein diet?

Diets that allow you to eat large quantities of high-protein, high-fat foods such as meat, eggs and whole milk while restricting your intake of carbohydrates periodically gain wide popularity. Part of their appeal is the rapid weight loss they can produce in a matter of days. Unfortunately, this rapid loss is due mostly to water excretion, not reduction of body fat. This water loss is caused by two basic metabolic adjustments your body makes when your diet omits carbohydrates. Initially, to keep up your blood sugar levels, your body consumes much of your glycogen, the carbohydrates that are stored in your liver and muscles. These carbohydrates are stored in combination with water, and their use results in a large water loss. After about 10 days on this kind of diet, your body increasingly draws on its fat for energy. However, because carbohydrates are necessary for the complete burning of fat, there is a build-up in the blood of ketone bodies, waste products from incomplete fat oxidation. The excretion of these waste products also uses up water, adding to your apparent weight loss.

A few days after you go off a high-protein diet, you will most probably regain the water you have lost as your body adjusts to the reintroduction of carbohydrates to your diet. Many doctors consider high-protein diets to be dangerous and believe that, through physiological mechanisms not completely understood, the metabolic changes these diets produce can cause serious health problems. In addition, the high fat content of many of these diets has been linked to an increased risk of certain kinds of cancer and cardiovascular problems.

Can you undertake a diet and exercise programme at any time?
Almost anyone can go on a diet and begin exercising. If you are extremely overweight, have high blood pressure or are diabetic, you should consult your doctor before trying to lose weight. Anyone who suffers from heart disease or any other condition that requires medical treatment should also seek a doctor's advice before embarking on a weight-loss regimen. Nursing mothers and pregnant women should avoid a restricted-calorie diet, except on the advice of their doctors.

How will this book help you control your weight?
It will give you a programme that is practical. The recipes in the following chapters are easy-to-make low-fat, high-carbohydrate dishes that provide an excellent foundation for a diet that allows gradual, permanent weight loss. The ingredients and cooking techniques in these recipes are designed to show you easy ways to cut down on dietary fat, yet prepare appetizing and nutritious dishes that supply generous portions. In addition, this book will guide you towards choosing proper between-meal snacks, dining out sensibly, exercising to burn more calories, and modifying other habits that have probably interfered with your weight control in the past. To start putting these elements together on a day-to-day basis, turn to the next page.

Diets That Don't Work

Despite the sheer number and seeming variety of popular diets, most of them fall into one of the categories shown on the right.

What all these diets promise is quick weight loss with relative ease. That they usually do not live up to expectations is obvious from the high failure rate of dieters: an estimated 75 to 95 per cent of people on a diet regain some or all of their lost weight within one or two years of going off their diets. Worse, many of these diets are dangerous because they rely on gimmicks that are deficient in essential vitamins and minerals.

A number of diets — especially those that combine high-protein or high-fat content with low-carbohydrate intake — produce a fluid loss that can fool dieters into thinking they are losing weight rapidly. In fact, the actual fat loss may be quite small, since the body cannot burn fat easily in the absence of carbohydrates. A by-product of this inefficient metabolism is a group of toxic waste products called ketone bodies, which stress, and can eventually damage, the body.

Nutritionists recommend that a reducing diet be nutritionally balanced, with the preponderance of calories coming from carbohydrates. Such a plan is not likely to cause a quick or dramatic weight loss, but the weight that is lost will be mainly excess fat and will stay off permanently if you exercise regularly and do not overeat. The guidelines for a healthy reducing diet, incorporating the recipes in this book, are spelled out on pages 34-39.

TYPE OF DIET	PREMISE	EFFECTS
FASTING 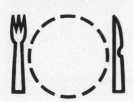	Complete abstinence from eating guarantees weight loss; your body's energy production is not offset by food intake but is supplied instead from the body's own tissues.	Initial weight loss is rapid, but much of the loss is from excretion of water and minerals. Metabolism soon slows to conserve energy, which diminishes rate of weight loss. Fasting also causes significant loss of muscle tissue. Heart arrhythmia may develop during refeeding after fasting. This is a drastic weight-loss measure that should only be attempted by the extremely obese, in a hospital, with medical supervision.
LIQUID PROTEIN 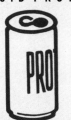	Dieter consumes only a special formula that is very low in calories and so loses weight. The protein content of the formula is supposed to keep the body from losing muscle tissue.	Weight loss may occur, but muscles are not spared as a result of consuming liquid protein. A prepackaged drink is also lacking in other essential nutrients. Possible side effects include nausea, diarrhoea and muscle cramps — and the formula may lack important minerals causing a deficiency that could result in a heart attack.
ONE FOOD 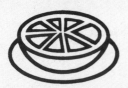	Consumption of one particular food or foods — such as grapefruit — causes your body to burn away extra fat.	In addition to being boring and hard to maintain, this diet is nutritionally deficient, since no one food contains all the nutrients necessary for good health. A diet in which fruit is the mainstay, for example, will be low in protein as well as in B vitamins, iron, zinc and calcium.
TIMETABLE 	Eating certain foods at specific times or in particular combinations speeds weight loss and improves your health by influencing digestion and absorption of calories and nutrients.	Combining foods in particular ways or eating them only at certain times has no proven effect on calorie utilization or nutrient retention. These diets often emphasize fruit and rice, making them too low in protein for optimal health.
HIGH PROTEIN, HIGH FAT 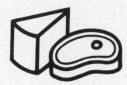	Restricting carbohydrate consumption while eating large helpings of meat and other fatty foods causes the body to burn fat.	Inclusion of rich foods makes these diets easy to stick to, but a high initial weight drop is due to water loss. In addition, the high-fat content may cause a rise in blood cholesterol, increasing the long-term risk of heart disease. Side effects include fatigue, bad breath and increased stress on liver and kidneys.
HIGH PROTEIN, LOW FAT 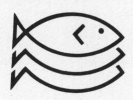	Restricting carbohydrate and fat intake while consuming mostly lean foods high in protein causes the body to burn fat.	Initial weight loss is water. This diet has the same side effects as the high-protein, high-fat diet.

How to Design Your Own Programme

Successfully setting your weight involves not only losing excess kilograms, but also maintaining that weight loss. The rest of this chapter will show you the steps to accomplishing this.

You will find guidelines on how to estimate your desirable weight; how to control your calorie intake and expenditure to reach that weight; how to plan low-calorie but appetizing menus; how to make sure that low-calorie meals are nutritionally balanced; and how to use a food and exercise diary as a tool for achieving your goals. You can then make use of the following chapters in the book to implement your programme.

Begin plotting your programme by reviewing the questions on the right. The answers will help you analyse why you may be having trouble with your weight and identify some of the habits, attitudes and behaviour traits you need to focus on to bring your weight under control.

Is your weight under control?

1 Do you think you look overweight?

Standing in front of a mirror can certainly give you a good indication of whether or not you are overweight. But some people have difficulty assessing their weight without the use of an objective guideline. Many of those who are overweight underestimate how much weight they should lose. Conversely, some people who are actually at their optimal weight think they should be thinner. Experts consider the tables on page 25 the best set of guidelines for showing how much you should weigh for optimal health and longevity.

If you do exceed the recommended weight for your age, height and sex, do not judge yourself too harshly. According to research, psychological suffering — including self-blame and feelings of inferiority — is among the most pervasive adverse effects of being overweight. Studies also show, however, that losing weight can help produce a positive self-image.

2 Have you lost weight and then regained it?

Many people are successful at losing weight, but keeping it off is another matter. More than three out of four people who lose weight gain it all back in less than a year — in most cases because they tried special diets that they stayed on for only a few weeks. The truth is, a gradual long-term approach to weight loss makes your programme more manageable and is far more realistic in terms of the results you should expect. Although you will probably see some changes in your weight and appearance very quickly using the guidelines in this book, it may take several months before substantial changes are evident.

3 Do you watch television while you eat?

Experts in behaviour modification recommend that meal times be free of competing activities so that your attention can be on your food. Distractions such as watching television can cause you to overeat without even realizing it because they lower your awareness of what you have consumed and how much.

4 Do you eat when you are anxious?

Depending on food to give you an emotional lift can contribute to overeating, especially if the foods you eat to make yourself feel better are high-calorie snack foods such as sweets or biscuits. Your snacks should be low-calorie, high-fibre foods, such as fruits and vegetables, that fill you up with relatively few calories.

Or, instead of focusing on eating as a mood lifter, substitute an activity such as aerobic exercise, which, studies show, can reduce stress and improve your mood at the same time that it burns calories.

5 **Do you share the misconception of most dieters about which foods are fattening?**

Generally, dieters overestimate the fattening effect of the carbohydrates they consume. By weight, sources of carbohydrates such as potatoes and pasta are not nearly as high in calories as the butter, creams and sauces that often accompany them. In fact, in a healthy and effective weight-loss programme about 55 to 60 per cent of the calories in your diet should come from carbohydrates — a guideline used in developing the recipes in this book.

6 **Do you drink alcohol every day?**

Alcohol provides no necessary nutrients, but it does contain 7 calories per gram, which is more than either carbohydrates or protein provide. For every 35 centilitre beer or 17.5 centilitre glass of wine you eliminate from your diet daily, you will save approximately 150 calories. Over a year those saved calories would be enough to account for more than seven lost kilograms. For tips on lower-calorie beverages, see the box on page 77.

7 **Can you recall what you ate yesterday?**

Without an accurate accounting of when and where you eat, you can easily miscalculate your present food intake, making it difficult to pinpoint the eating habits that are causing you to gain weight. Using a diary such as the one on page 41 provides a tangible record. You should keep this diary to analyse your current eating patterns before you start your weight-loss programme and then use it to record your progress as you lose weight.

How fast should you lose weight?

You should lose up to 1 kilogram per week. Any loss greater than that will probably be the result of a highly restrictive programme that you will not be able to maintain for very long. An extremely rapid weight loss is usually from large water losses rather than loss of fat. As soon as you go off a diet that causes water loss, you quickly regain those kilograms of liquid. Furthermore, if you are losing more than 1 kilogram a week through dieting, you are probably not getting the nutrients you need to stay healthy.

To obtain a realistic picture of your actual weight loss, you should only weigh yourself once a week. This should preferably be first thing in the morning, before breakfast and before getting dressed. Always use the same set of scales. If it is not possible for you to follow this early morning regime, at least make sure you always weigh yourself at the same time of day and on the same scales. Remove your coat, shoes and heavy jewellery first. Allow about 1 kilogram for indoor clothing and subtract this from the total.

For each half-kilogram you shed, you need to create a deficit of approximately 3,500 calories between the calories you eat and the calories you use up in activity. Therefore, to lose about half a kilogram per week, you need to use up 500 more calories per day in physical activity than you consume in your food. The calorie charts for foods and activities in this book will guide you towards creating this calorie deficit.

Your Optimal Weight

The most accurate assessment of your ideal weight takes into account the composition of your body — how much of your weight is lean body mass (muscle and bone) and how much is body fat. For optimum health, body fat should constitute no more than 20 per cent of total body weight for men or 30 per cent for women. However, to determine body composition accurately requires both professional analysis and sophisticated equipment. Much simpler and more convenient guidelines to optimal weight are the tables of acceptable weights recommended by the Fogarty Conference, U.S.A. in 1979 and by the United Kingdom's Royal College of Physicians in 1983, which were published in Britain by the National Advisory Committee on Nutrition Education in 1983.

The tables, reproduced on the opposite page, established a healthy weight range for each height and sex group based on the statistics for longevity collated by life insurance companies. People who fell within the desirable weight range had lived for significantly longer than people on either side.

The weight tables do not include any upward adjustment for age, since there are no good reasons for a person to weigh more as he gets older. Indeed, since the amount of muscle (which is denser than fat) decreases with age, body weight should ideally decline with advancing years. Nor do the tables include any adjustment for frame size, since people with larger bones do not necessarily have denser bones, which would give a markedly greater body weight. True, a fine-limbed person ought to weigh rather less than a thickset person. As a fairly large weight range is given for each height, however, this should take into account any significant differences in frame size. A person with a petite physique ought to aim for an ideal weight at the lower end of the range, whereas a person of the same height but with a larger physique could quite satisfactorily weigh in at the top of the range.

An alternative way of gauging your weight is to calculate your Body Mass Index (BMI). To work it out, divide your weight in kilograms by your height in metres squared. The normal acceptable range of this measurement is 20.1 to 25.0 units for males and 18.7 to 23.8 for females, irrespective of whether they are lightly or heavily built. In general, people within these ranges are more free from disease and have lower mortality rates than people outside. Anyone over the limit of 25.0 units for men or 23.8 for women is tending towards obesity. The only exceptions are athletes and body builders, whose extra muscle may tip their BMI over the normal range.

Desirable Weights

HEIGHT without shoes (m)	MEN Weight without clothes (kg)			WOMEN Weight without clothes (kg)		
	Acceptable average	Acceptable weight range	Obese	Acceptable average	Acceptable weight range	Obese
1.45				46.0	42-53	64
1.48				46.5	42-54	65
1.50				47.0	43-55	66
1.52				48.5	44-57	68
1.54				49.5	44-58	70
1.56				50.4	45-58	70
1.58	55.8	51-64	77	51.3	46-59	71
1.60	57.6	52-65	78	52.6	48-61	73
1.62	58.6	53-66	79	54.0	49-62	74
1.64	59.6	54-67	80	55.4	50-64	77
1.66	60.6	55-69	83	56.8	51-65	78
1.68	61.7	56-71	85	58.1	52-66	79
1.70	63.5	58-73	88	60.0	53-67	80
1.72	65.0	59-74	89	61.3	55-69	83
1.74	66.5	60-75	90	62.6	56-70	84
1.76	68.0	62-77	92	64.0	58-72	86
1.78	69.4	64-79	95	65.3	59-74	89
1.80	71.0	65-80	96			
1.82	72.6	66-82	98			
1.84	74.2	67-84	101			
1.86	75.8	69-86	103			
1.88	77.6	71-88	106			
1.90	79.3	73-90	108			
1.92	81.0	75-93	112			
BMI*	22.0	20.1-25.0	30.0	20.8	18.7-23.8	28.6

*Body mass index = weight in kilograms/height^2 in metres

Calorie Trade-Offs

330 CALORIES

 =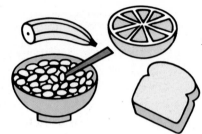

3 breakfast sausages
(30 grams each)

25 centilitres skimmed milk

½ grapefruit (100 grams)
½ banana (90 grams)
1 slice brown
toast (30 grams)
1 teaspoon sugar
30 grams puffed wheat cereal

100 CALORIES

 =

½ head iceberg lettuce (200 grams)
60 grams mushrooms
60 grams carrot
90 grams tomato
60 grams cucumber slices

1 tablespoon bottled
French dressing

10 grams onion slices

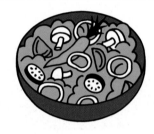

460 CALORIES

 =

1 hamburger (120 grams)
1 slice cheese (30 grams)
1 hamburger bun (45 grams)

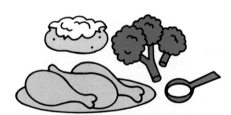

3 skinless roasted chicken
drumsticks (175 grams meat)
100 grams cooked broccoli
1 baked potato (200 grams)
1 tablespoon
plain low-fat yogurt

265 CALORIES

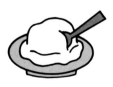 =

100 grams dairy
ice cream

1 oatmeal biscuit (15 grams)
15 centilitres plain
low-fat yogurt
100 grams strawberries
1 teaspoon sugar

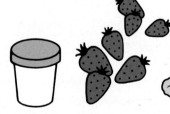

The Calories You Eat

Eliminating dietary calories to the point where you will lose weight does not require eating minuscule amounts of food or counting calories obsessively. The most efficient way to reduce your calorie intake is to eat less fat.

By weight, dietary fat contains more than twice the calories of protein and carbohydrates — nine calories per gram compared with four calories per gram of the other two major nutrients. This fact explains why 100 grams of peanuts, which contain 49 grams of fat, have about four times as many calories as 100 grams of cooked kidney beans, which contain only a trace of fat. Likewise, the dishes on the left side of the illustration opposite boast a high fat content which means that they pack a lot of calories into relatively small portions. The dishes on the right, by contrast, are low in fat and so allow you to eat more food for the same number of calories.

In the average British diet, about 40 per cent of the total calories consumed are from fat. One major contributor of this fat is red meat. But almost half of all dietary fat comes from vegetable oils, shortening and lard, which are used during cooking and baking or added at the table in spreads and dressings. Dairy products and eggs, whose fat content is often highly concentrated, contribute another 15 per cent.

Generally, the fat in your diet should supply 30 per cent or less of your total calories. Take the first step towards a low-fat diet by assessing the fat content of your current diet. Use the chart on the next two pages — it not only shows calorie values for common foods, but also indicates what percentage of those calories come from fat.

The best way to keep a weight-control diet healthy and relatively satisfying is to replace fatty foods with complex carbohydrates — the starches in grains, cereals, pulses and vegetables. These foods contain far fewer calories than an equivalent amount of red meat but contain some vitamins and minerals that meat lacks. You do not have to eliminate meat from your diet entirely, but you should choose the leanest cuts and eat it no more than once a day, in portions of no more than 90 to 120 grams per serving. Or, better still, eat lean fish or white meat poultry with the skin removed.

Along with cutting back on meat, you should make other low-calorie substitutions to trim your intake of fat and also of refined sugar, another substantial source of calories. Use such dairy products as skimmed and semi-skimmed milk, and low-fat cheeses and yogurt; avoid fried foods and canned foods packed in oil; eat fruits for desserts and snacks rather than cakes, biscuits and other items high in refined sugar as well as fat. The recipes in this book provide an excellent way of incorporating these strategies into your eating plan.

The key to maintaining a low-calorie eating regimen is to take a gradual approach. If you use the recipes and tips in this book steadily to cut a small number of calories from your diet each day, you will soon notice results. Even a daily reduction of a mere 200 or 300 calories — which you can achieve just by cutting out the cream in your coffee and the mayonnaise on your sandwich, for example — will allow you to lose half a kilogram in less than two weeks. Changing your diet in small stages keeps you from feeling deprived, which in turn makes it more likely that you will stick with your new eating habits.

A Guide to Calorie Consumption

Food (per 100 g/3½ oz)		Calories	% Fat*	Food (per 100 g/3½ oz)		Calories	% Fat*
Almonds		565	85	**Celery**	raw	8	Trace
Apples		46	Trace		boiled	5	Trace
Apple juice		49	Trace	**Cereals**	bran flakes, sugared	302	3
Apple pie		369	38		cornflakes	368	4
Apricots	fresh	28	Trace		porridge, made with water	44	18
	dried	182	Trace		puffed rice	372	5
Asparagus		18	Trace		puffed wheat	325	4
Avocado pear		223	90		muesli	368	18
Bacon	back, grilled	405	75	**Cheese**	Camembert	300	70
	back, fried	465	79		cottage	96	38
Bananas		79	3		Cheddar	406	74
Bean sprouts		35	Trace		cream	439	97
Beans	French, boiled	7	Trace		Danish blue	355	74
Beef	minced, stewed	229	60		Parmesan	408	66
	rump steak, lean grilled	168	32		ricotta, low-fat	145	52
	topside, lean roast	156	25	**Cherries**	fresh	47	Trace
Beer	draught	32	Trace	**Chicken**	white meat, roast, no skin	142	25
	lager	29	Trace		dark meat, roast, no skin	155	40
Beetroot	boiled	44	Trace	**Courgettes**		25	Trace
Biscuits	cream crackers	440	33	**Cream**	double	447	97
	crispbread, rye	321	6		single	212	90
	digestive, plain	471	39	**Cucumber**		10	Trace
	digestive, chocolate	493	44	**Dates**	dried	248	Trace
	ginger nuts	456	30	**Egg**	boiled	147	67
	shortbread	504	46		fried	232	76
	water biscuits	440	26		poached	155	68
Blackberries	fresh	29	Trace		scrambled	246	83
Black-eyed beans	raw	343	2	**Fish**	cod, fried in batter	199	47
Blueberries	fresh	62	Trace		cod, steamed	83	10
Bread	white	233	7		crab, boiled	127	37
	wholemeal	216	11		haddock, steamed	98	7
Broccoli	tops, boiled	18	Trace		halibut, steamed	131	27
Brussels sprouts	boiled	18	Trace		oysters	51	16
Buns and pastries	currant bun	302	23		plaice, steamed	93	18
	doughnut	349	41		prawns, boiled	107	15
	éclair	376	57		salmon, steamed	197	59
	jam tart	384	35		scallops, steamed	105	12
	mince pie	435	43		sole, fried	216	54
	scone	371	35		sole, steamed	91	9
Butter		740	100		trout, steamed	135	30
Cabbage	raw	22	Trace		tuna, canned in oil	289	69
	cooked	15	Trace	**Grapefruit**		22	Trace
Cake	brownie	451	57	**Grapefruit juice**	sweetened	38	Trace
	fruit cake	332	30		unsweetened	31	Trace
	gingerbread	373	30	**Grapes**		61	Trace
	Madeira	393	39	**Haricot beans**	boiled	93	5
	sponge, with fat	464	51	**Honey**		288	Trace
	sponge, genoise	301	20	**Ice cream**	dairy	167	36
Carrots	raw	23	Trace	**Jams and preserves**		261	0
	cooked	19	Trace	**Lamb**	cutlets, grilled, lean and fat	370	75
Cashew nuts		561	73		cutlets, grilled, lean only	222	50
Cauliflower	raw	13	Trace		leg, roast, lean and fat	266	61
	cooked	9	Trace		leg, roast, lean only	191	38

Food (per 100 g/3½ oz)		Calories	% Fat*
Lemons		15	0
Lentils	cooked	99	5
Lettuce		12	Trace
Liver	lamb's, raw	90	27
	lamb's, fried	155	37
Macaroni	cooked	117	5
Margarine		730	100
Marrow	boiled	7	Trace
Mayonnaise		718	99
Melon	cantaloupe	24	Trace
	honeydew	21	Trace
	watermelon	21	Trace
Milk	whole	65	53
	semi-skimmed	49	37
	skimmed	33	3
Mushrooms	raw	13	Trace
	fried	210	22
Oil	corn, olive or sunflower	899	100
Onions	raw	23	Trace
	fried	345	87
Oranges	fresh	35	Trace
Orange juice	pure	38	Trace
Pancake		307	48
Peaches	fresh	37	Trace
	canned in syrup	87	Trace
Peanuts		570	77
Peanut butter		623	78
Pears	fresh	29	Trace
	canned in syrup	77	Trace
Pickled cucumber	dill	8	Trace
Pineapple	raw	46	Trace
	canned in syrup	77	Trace
Pizza	cheese and tomato	234	44
Plums	fresh	38	Trace
Popcorn	plain	383	Trace
Pork	loin chop, grilled, lean and fat	332	66
	loin chop, grilled, lean only	226	43
	leg, roast, lean and fat	286	62
	leg, roast, lean only	185	34
Potatoes	baked, with skin	105	Trace
	boiled	80	Trace
	chips	253	39
	crisps	533	61
Pretzels		415	11.5
Prunes		161	Trace

Food (per 100 g/3½ oz)		Calories	% Fat*
Pumpkin		15	Trace
Raisins		246	Trace
Raspberries	fresh	25	Trace
Rice	white, raw	361	2
	white, boiled	123	2
	brown, raw	357	7
Salad dressing	French	658	99
Sausage	beef, grilled	265	59
	pork, grilled	318	70
	frankfurter	274	82
	salami	491	83
	liver sausage	310	78
Soup	chicken noodle	20	13
	lentil	99	34
	oxtail	44	35
	tomato, cream of	55	54
	vegetable	37	17
Spaghetti	raw	378	2
	boiled	117	2
Spinach	raw	26	10
Spirits	gin, rum, vodka, brandy, whisky	222	0
Strawberries	fresh	26	Trace
Sugar	white or brown	394	Trace
Sweet pepper		15	Trace
Sweet potato	boiled	85	6
Syrup	golden	298	0
	blackstrap molasses	257	0
Tomato		14	Trace
Tomato ketchup		98	Trace
Tomato purée		67	Trace
Turkey	white meat, roast, no skin	132	10
	dark meat, roast, no skin	148	25
Veal	cutlet, fried	215	34
Venison	roast	198	29
Vinegar		4	0
Walnuts		525	88
Wine	red, dry	68	0
	white, dry	66	0
	white, sweet	94	0
Yeast	baker's compressed	53	7
	dried	169	8
Yogurt	Greek, plain	140	64
	low-fat, plain	52	17
	low-fat, flavoured	81	1

Caloric and fat content can vary depending upon methods of food processing and analysis.

*The figures for fat content indicate the percentage of calories that are derived from fat, not the percentage of fat by weight. ("Trace" means that the percentage of fat is nutritionally negligible.) An effective weight-loss programme should limit foods that derive more than 30 per cent of their calories from fat.

The Calories You Burn

It is far more difficult to lose weight permanently if you are sedentary than if you are physically active. A number of studies have found that many obese people do not eat significantly more than thinner ones, but the obese are much less active. Similarly, the kilogram or two of weight that many adults put on each year when they reach middle age may be due to decreasing physical activity rather than a change in eating patterns. Studies indicate that adults who are physically active throughout their lives maintain a desirable weight.

Researchers have also confirmed that exercise preserves and builds up muscle tissue. Firm muscles not only improve your appearance, but also aid in weight loss because added muscle, unlike body fat, continually burns calories. Moreover, some evidence suggests that vigorous exercise helps to suppress appetite rather than stimulate it, as many people believe.

A crucial part of any weight-loss programme, therefore, is adding activities to your daily life that will substantially increase calorie expenditure. To do this is not easy: labour-saving devices at work and at home contribute to a sedentary lifestyle. The illustrations opposite show substitutions you can make to replace sedentary routines with more strenuous ones. For example, a brisk 20-minute walk burns up about 120 calories for a 68-kilogram person. If you did this five days a week for a year rather than travel in a car, you would expend an extra 23,500 calories — equivalent to a weight loss of over 3 kilograms.

One group of researchers has estimated that office workers could lose up to 7 kilograms a year and homemakers 9 kilograms a year by substituting more active behaviour for their normal sedentary routines. The calorie chart given on pages 32-33 will give you some idea of the calories expended for a wide range of daily activities.

The surest way to increase calorie output significantly is with a programme of regular exercise. In the following chapters, you will find exercise tips and routines preceding each recipe section. The exercises range from moderate to strenuous levels of exertion, and some of them, particularly the exercises in Chapter Three, are designed to build muscle as you shed weight. To burn off significant amounts of fat, your exercise must be aerobic — meaning that it supplies oxygen to major muscle groups for an extended period. Such exercises, which usually utilize the large muscles of the legs, include cycling, running, brisk walking, skipping, aerobic movement, certain callisthenic routines and various racket sports. The chart on page 115 will help you to choose an exercise and develop a regimen.

As with changing your diet, you are far more likely to make exercise a permanent part of your life if you ease into it gradually. Overexerting yourself can cause you to become fatigued quickly or to injure yourself, and either one increases the likelihood that you will give up exercise. If you combine exercising consistently with a reduction in your calorie intake, you will not only take weight off but keep it off.

Getting Active

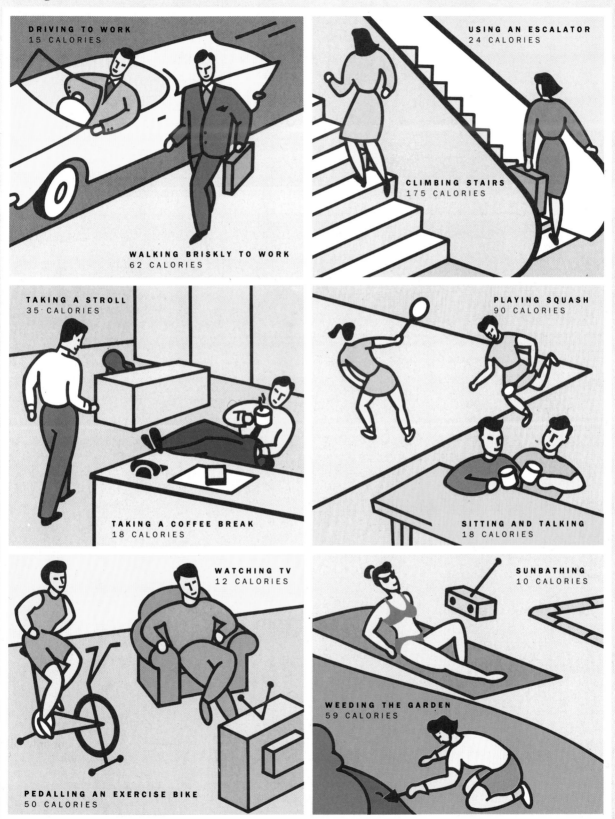

DRIVING TO WORK
15 CALORIES

USING AN ESCALATOR
24 CALORIES

CLIMBING STAIRS
175 CALORIES

WALKING BRISKLY TO WORK
62 CALORIES

TAKING A STROLL
35 CALORIES

PLAYING SQUASH
90 CALORIES

TAKING A COFFEE BREAK
18 CALORIES

SITTING AND TALKING
18 CALORIES

WATCHING TV
12 CALORIES

SUNBATHING
10 CALORIES

WEEDING THE GARDEN
59 CALORIES

PEDALLING AN EXERCISE BIKE
50 CALORIES

Calorie counts are for 10 minutes of activity

A Guide to Calorie Expenditure

Activity	Calories burned per minute (by body weight)			Activity	Calories burned per minute (by body weight)		
	50 kg	68 kg	85 kg		50 kg	68 kg	85 kg
Chopping wood with an axe, fast	14.8	20.2	25.6	Forking straw bales	6.9	9.4	11.9
Running, level ground, 5.5 min metric mile*	14.4	19.7	24.9	Riding, galloping	6.8	9.3	11.8
Skin diving, considerable motion	13.8	18.8	23.8	Aerobic dance, intense	6.7	9.2	11.6
Skiing, cross-country, uphill	13.7	18.6	23.6	Running, horizontal, 11.5 min metric mile*	6.7	9.2	11.6
Running, 6 min metric mile*	12.6	17.1	21.7	Hockey	6.7	9.1	11.5
Running, 7 min metric mile*	11.4	15.5	19.6	Football	6.6	9.0	11.4
Boxing	11.1	15.1	19.1	Felling trees	6.6	9.0	11.4
Squash	10.6	14.4	18.3	Climbing hills with 4 kg load	6.4	8.8	11.1
Running, 8 min metric mile*	10.4	14.1	17.9	Swimming, crawl, slow	6.4	8.7	11.0
Skipping, 145 jumps per minute	9.8	13.4	17.0	Digging	6.3	8.6	10.9
Judo	9.7	13.3	16.8	Sawing by hand	6.1	8.3	10.5
Running, 9 min metric mile*	9.6	13.1	16.6	Swimming, sidestroke	6.1	8.3	10.5
Carrying logs	9.3	12.7	16.0	Climbing hills with no load	6.0	8.2	10.4
Racketball	8.9	12.1	15.3	Skiing, cross-country, moderate speed	5.9	8.1	10.3
Skipping, 125 jumps per minute	8.8	12.0	15.3	Lawn mowing	5.6	7.6	9.7
Treading water, fast	8.5	11.6	14.6	Riding, trotting	5.5	7.5	9.5
Cycling, racing	8.4	11.5	14.6	Planting by hand	5.4	7.4	9.4
Swimming, backstroke	8.4	11.5	14.6	Scrubbing floors	5.4	7.4	9.4
Snowshoeing, soft snow	8.3	11.3	14.3	Tennis	5.4	7.4	9.4
Skipping, 80 jumps per minute	8.2	11.2	14.1	Shovelling coal	5.4	7.3	9.3
Skipping, 70 jumps per minute	8.1	11.0	14.0	Aerobic dance, medium	5.1	7.0	8.9
Swimming, breaststroke, fast	8.1	11.0	14.0	Cycling, leisure 15 km/h	5.0	6.8	8.6
Swimming, crawl, fast	7.8	10.6	13.4	Skiing, soft snow	4.9	6.7	8.4
Climbing hills with 20 kg load	7.3	10.0	12.7	Badminton	4.8	6.6	8.4
Digging trenches	7.2	9.9	12.5	Weight training, circuit training	4.6	6.3	7.9
Skiing, cross-country, walking	7.1	9.7	12.3	Hoeing	4.5	6.2	7.8
Marching, rapid	7.1	9.7	12.2	Cricket, bowling	4.5	6.1	7.8
Climbing hills with 10 kg load	7.0	9.5	12.1	Stacking firewood	4.4	6.0	7.6
Basketball	6.9	9.4	11.9	Weight lifting, free weights	4.3	5.9	7.4
Boxing, sparring	6.9	9.4	11.9	Shovelling grain	4.2	5.8	7.3

* metric mile = 1,500 metres

Rating Activities

The chart above lists activities and exercises by the number of calories they use up, starting with activities that burn the most. Since almost all energy production by the body uses oxygen, researchers can assess an activity's calorie value by evaluating how much oxygen is used when performing it. You do not use all of the oxygen in the air you breathe in, no matter how demanding the activity you are doing, and therefore your exhaled air contains some oxygen. In order to determine the amount of oxygen an activity requires, researchers collect a subject's exhaled air in a rubber bag during an activity and they then compare the amount of oxygen in this exhaled air with the amount of oxygen in the ambient air. The difference in the percentages of oxygen enables the

Activity	Calories burned per minute (by body weight)			Activity	Calories burned per minute (by body weight)		
	50 kg	68 kg	85 kg		50 kg	68 kg	85 kg
Golf	4.2	5.8	7.3	Cooking	2.4	3.3	4.1
Cricket, batting	4.1	5.6	7.2	Wallpapering	2.4	3.3	4.1
Walking, normal pace, fields and hills	4.1	5.6	7.1	Violin playing, sitting	2.2	3.1	3.9
Walking, normal pace, grass	4.0	5.5	7.0	Sewing by machine	2.2	3.1	3.9
Walking, normal pace, tarmac road	4.0	5.4	6.9	Canoeing	2.2	3.0	3.8
Plastering	3.9	5.3	6.7	Billiards	2.1	2.9	3.6
House painting, exteriors	3.8	5.2	6.6	Riding, walking	2.0	2.8	3.5
Walking, normal pace, ploughed field	3.8	5.2	6.6	Cello playing, sitting	2.0	2.8	3.5
Sawing, power	3.7	5.1	6.5	Driving harvester	2.0	2.7	3.4
Weeding	3.6	4.9	6.2	Piano playing, sitting	2.0	2.7	3.4
Table tennis	3.4	4.6	5.9	Conducting music	1.9	2.7	3.4
Gymnastics	3.3	4.5	5.7	Bookbinding	1.9	2.6	3.3
Playing drums, sitting	3.3	4.5	5.7	Driving tractor	1.8	2.5	3.2
Archery	3.2	4.4	5.6	Drawing, standing	1.8	2.4	3.1
Cycling, 9 km/h	3.2	4.4	5.5	Flute playing, sitting	1.7	2.4	3.0
Scraping paint	3.1	4.3	5.4	Accordion playing, sitting	1.6	2.2	2.8
Fishing	3.1	4.2	5.3	Woodwind playing, sitting	1.6	2.2	2.8
Food shopping	3.1	4.2	5.3	Sewing by hand	1.6	2.2	2.8
Mopping floors	3.1	4.2	5.3	Trumpet playing, standing	1.5	2.1	2.7
Treading water, normal	3.1	4.2	5.3	Typing, manual	1.5	2.1	2.7
Croquet	2.9	4.0	5.1	Horn playing, sitting	1.4	2.0	2.5
Cleaning	2.9	3.9	5.0	Writing, sitting	1.4	2.0	2.5
Window cleaning	2.9	3.9	5.0	Standing still	1.3	1.8	2.3
Milking cows by hand	2.7	3.7	4.7	Typing, electric	1.3	1.8	2.3
Raking	2.7	3.7	4.7	Card playing	1.2	1.7	2.2
Organ playing, sitting	2.6	3.6	4.6	Eating, sitting	1.1	1.6	2.0
Carpentry	2.6	3.5	4.5	Milking cows by machine	1.1	1.6	2.0
Welding	2.6	3.5	4.5	Knitting	1.1	1.5	1.9
Dancing, ballroom	2.5	3.5	4.4	Lying still	1.1	1.5	1.9
Volleyball	2.5	3.4	4.3	Sitting still	1.0	1.4	1.8

researchers to calculate how many calories were expended.

For any activity, however, the energy cost is affected by a multitude of factors that vary from person to person. For example, as the chart indicates, the heavier you are, the more calories you will burn performing many activities. This is because the added kilograms contribute to the effort of any movement. Your level of conditioning, the temperature and the humidity of the air and how efficiently you perform an activity also affect calorie expenditure.

Although the values are approximate rather than precise measurements, you can use this chart to estimate the number of calories you burn during exertion. Choosing the more energetic activities will aid you in reducing your weight.

Planning Your Meals

When you take the responsibility for planning your own meals, rather than following a set diet, you can choose foods that please your palate and satisfy your hunger while meeting your calorie limitations and fulfilling your nutritional needs. Although you should be aware of the calorie content of foods, you do not have to count every calorie in order to lose weight. Just keep in mind these three basic principles: eat foods that are low in fat and high in complex carbohydrates, eat modest portions and eat a variety of foods.

The menus on these two pages — intended as examples, not blueprints — show you how to apply these principles. Each menu totals 1,500 to 1,600 calories daily, which nutritionists consider the minimum for most people on a weight-loss programme that includes exercise.

These menus combine recipes from this book with other foods to lend variety to the meals and to meet nutritional requirements; however, any eating plan that restricts your calories also limits your intake of vitamins and minerals. On page 38, you will find a set of guidelines to ensure that your weight-loss programme stays nutritionally balanced.

Weekday breakfasts have to be fast: make a batch of whole-grain muffins and freeze them individually. In the morning, heat one in the toaster. For snacks at work, eat low-fat savoury biscuits rather than vending-machine fare or other high-calorie foods. Skimmed or semi-skimmed milk, with calcium and B vitamins, can be added to snacks.

For lunch, a salad you make the night before can be taken to work in an insulated container. At afternoon break time, keep your hunger pangs at bay with a low-calorie spread and vegetables.

After work, it takes just minutes to prepare a salad and stir fry precooked chicken and broccoli (using a combination of chicken stock and oil to save calories).

WEEKDAY

	Calories
Breakfast	
Cornmeal-Cheese Muffin with herbed ricotta spread (page 54)	335
Coffee or tea (optional)	
Mid-morning snack	
6 Rye-Cheese Biscuits (page 71)	85
20 centilitres semi-skimmed milk	95
Lunch	
Florida Halibut Salad (page 92)	305
20 centilitres semi-skimmed milk	95
Medium-sized peach	40
Mid-afternoon snack	
White Bean-Chèvre Spread (page 106)	190
Dinner	
Large spinach-mushroom salad with 3 tablespoons yogurt-orange juice dressing	80
90 grams poached chicken breast and 120 grams blanched broccoli, stir fried with spring onions and ginger in a non-stick frying pan using 1 teaspoon of oil and 2 tablespoons chicken stock; served with 120 grams cooked rice	340
total	1,565

SPECIAL OCCASION

	Calories
Breakfast	
30 grams vitamin-mineral fortified cereal	100
12.5 centilitres semi-skimmed milk	55
100 grams sliced strawberries	30
Mid-morning snack	
20 centilitres low-fat vanilla yogurt	100
Coffee or tea (optional)	
Lunch	
Curried Vegetable Soup (page 91)	265
12.5 centilitres semi-skimmed milk	55
Mid-afternoon snack	
20 centilitres low-fat vanilla yogurt	100
Dinner (restaurant)	
Tossed salad of leaf lettuce, cos lettuce, cucumber and tomatoes; request oil and vinegar on the side and use no more than 2 teaspoons of oil	105
175 grams lean roast leg of lamb 120 grams herbed rice 90 grams steamed asparagus 1 teaspoon butter	450
20 centilitres red wine	85
Small slice chocolate layer cake	230
total	1,575

Although you should try to focus on the non-food aspects of celebrations, advance planning permits you to indulge in foods you would otherwise avoid.

Eating fewer calories earlier in the day allows you to "bank" some calories for a glass of wine and/or a dessert at dinner. Just be sure that your breakfast, lunch and snack foods supply the required vitamins and minerals.

The restaurant dinner here begins with a salad — a good start because it takes the edge off your appetite. Eat slowly, and do not feel obliged to finish oversized restaurant portions. Try to stop when you are almost full: you can then go ahead and enjoy a modest dessert.

WEEKEND

	Calories
Pre-exercise snack	
Strawberry-Orange Milk Shake (page 52)	125
Pineapple-Oat Muffin (page 63)	185
Breakfast	
Gingerbread Brown-Rice Griddle Cake (page 64)	245
Lunch	
Tomato filled with 60 grams water-packed tuna, 2 tablespoons low-fat yogurt, 2 tablespoons chopped celery; served on 100 grams spinach leaves	115
20 centilitres semi-skimmed milk	95
10 dried apricot halves	85
Mid-afternoon snack	
Fruit-Bowl Drink (page 104)	100
Dinner	
Greek Salad (page 121)	170
Lentil Minestrone (page 128)	285
Lime Bavarian (page 100)	140
total	1,545

At weekends, when you have extra time, you may plan a longer workout than you can fit in during the week.

You may want a snack before you exercise; if so, choose the shake or the muffin — or both. After your workout enjoy a leisurely breakfast of griddle cakes.

Lunch is easy and low in calories but provides substantial protein, calcium and iron. The fruit drink refreshes you during the afternoon and contains plenty of vitamins A and C.

You probably have more time to cook at weekends, so this dinner is a bit more elaborate than the usual weekday meal. A large salad and a hearty soup are followed by a dessert that you can make in advance and chill until dinner time.

Low-Calorie Cooking

The recipes in this volume are designed to fit a menu plan of 1,500 to 1,600 calories per day: 300 to 400 calories contained in each of three meals, and about 300 to 400 calories divided between two snacks. The recipes were created to provide a variety of flavours and textures and to include dishes from a wide range of cuisines. The example below, a main-dish salad, highlights some of the ways these recipes provide generous amounts of food while limiting calories through the careful choice of ingredients and the use of cooking techniques that require little or no fat. You can also use these principles to help you choose recipes from many other sources to suit a low-calorie, low-fat diet.

A The recipe headnote highlights a particularly important nutrient or a low-calorie ingredient that is contained in the recipe.

B These recipes include a minimal amount of meat — enough for good nutrition, but not so much as to make the dishes overly high in fat and protein. In this recipe, 250 grams of chicken for four servings is supplemented with a large amount of high-carbohydrate vegetables. Removing the chicken skin before cooking is an example of a technique that cuts fat content — here, by about 50 per cent.

C Wherever possible, the use of oil in these recipes is limited, since oils are 100 per cent fat. In this case, chicken stock substitutes as the main basis for the salad dressing, which keeps the oil and fat content down.

D Many conventional recipes depend on high-fat ingredients to provide flavour. In the recipes in this book, herbs are used to heighten flavour without adding calories.

E Throughout the book, vegetables are used in generous amounts: they are very filling because of their high fibre content but low in calories. (All the vegetables in one serving of this dish add up to just 65 calories.)

F The ingredients for these recipes are chosen for their nutritional content as well as for their taste and low calories. The mango used here has only 135 calories, but supplies more than the RDA of vitamins A and C. It also contains generous amounts of potassium and niacin.

G Techniques such as poaching, which keeps chicken and fish moist and tender, are used instead of methods such as frying, which adds fat.

H Prepare your vegetables as close as possible to the serving time to preserve taste and nutrients.

I The calorie counts for main dishes in this book are below 400; for snacks, the average serving does not exceed 200 calories.

J The percentages in the nutrition charts refer to carbohydrates, protein and fat as ratios of the total calorie count, not of the weight of the ingredients (which is given in grams). This dish, like the others in this book, conforms to National Advisory Committee on Nutrition Education guidelines for high-carbohydrate/low-fat eating *(see page 38).*

K The calcium and iron listings are designed to help you calculate your intake of these two important minerals. The chart on page 39 will help you identify sources for calcium and iron to ensure that you get enough.

L The recipes in this book keep salt to a minimum and limit high-sodium ingredients.

GREEN SALAD WITH CHICKEN AND MANGOES

A *You can get half of your daily requirement of niacin from the chicken and mangoes in this salad.*

B 250 g (8 oz) boneless skinless
   chicken breast
   12.5 cl (4 fl oz) low-sodium
   chicken stock
C 4 tablespoons lemon juice
   2 tablespoons olive oil
D 1 teaspoon finely chopped fresh
   tarragon, or ¼ teaspoon dried
   tarragon, crumbled
   ¼ teaspoon salt

¼ teaspoon black pepper
1 cos lettuce
2 bunches watercress
300 g (10 oz) sweet red
   peppers, diced
E 75 g (2½ oz) shredded
   red cabbage
100 g (3½ oz) spring onions,
   finely chopped
4 mangoes, peeled and diced F

I CALORIES per serving	325
J 54% Carbohydrate	47 g
24% Protein	21g
22% Fat	9g
CALCIUM	241 mg
IRON	4 mg
L SODIUM	236 mg

K

G Place the chicken in a small saucepan, add cold water to cover and bring to the boil over medium-high heat. Reduce the heat so that the water simmers and poach the chicken for 5 minutes, or just until cooked through; transfer it to a plate and set aside to cool to room temperature.

For the dressing, whisk together the stock, lemon juice, oil, tarragon, salt and pepper in a small bowl; set aside. Wash the lettuce and watercress. Tear the lettuce into bite-sized pieces, trim the watercress and combine the greens in a H large bowl. Add the peppers, cabbage and spring onions and toss well.

Cut the chicken diagonally into thin slices. Whisk the dressing briefly to reblend it. Add the chicken, mangoes and dressing to the salad and toss gently. Divide the salad among four plates and serve.   Makes 4 servings

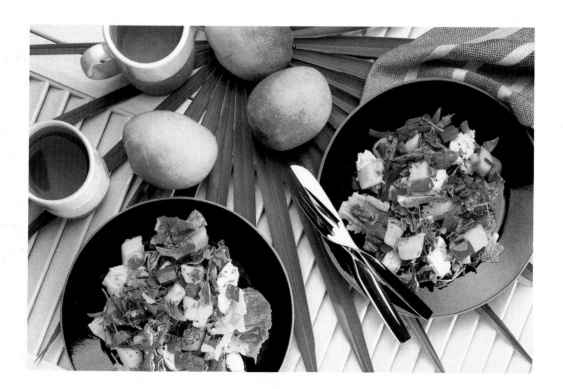

Nutritional Guidelines

The nutrition charts that accompany the recipes in this book include the number of calories per serving, the number of grams of fat, carbohydrate and protein in a serving, and the percentage of calories derived from each of these nutrients. The charts also provide the amount of calcium, iron and sodium per serving. Although the number of calories taken in and expended is what actually determines whether you will gain or lose weight, the fat, carbohydrate and protein content of your diet is most important to your health. Britain's National Advisory Committee on Nutrition Education recommends that no more than 30 per cent of the calories in your diet come from fat, that around 11 per cent come from protein and hence 55 to 60 per cent come from carbohydrates. A gram of fat equals nine calories, whereas a gram of protein or carbohydrate equals four calories; therefore, if you eat 1,500 calories a day, you should consume approximately 50 grams of fat, 220 grams of carbohydrate and no more than 45 grams of protein daily.

◆ The fats you consume should be mainly monounsaturated and polyunsaturated fats, such as those found in most vegetable oils. The saturated fat found in meat, high-fat dairy products, palm oil and coconut oil is associated with the formation of cholesterol in the blood, and elevated blood cholesterol levels play a significant role in heart disease.

◆ Most of the carbohydrates you eat should be complex (such as those found in grains, beans and starchy vegetables) rather than simple (the sugars common in highly processed foods). Fruits contain fructose, a simple carbohydrate, but they also contain vitamins, minerals and fibre.

◆ Turn to low-fat protein sources: substitute chicken or fish for red meat and use vegetable protein sources such as grain products and beans. The average British diet supplies more protein than most people require, so if you eat less meat, you will probably not be lacking for protein.

◆ A low-calorie diet may reduce your intake of four nutrients — calcium, iron, niacin and thiamine — that are essential to good health, as explained below. The box opposite lists low-calorie sources for these nutrients and gives the Recommended Daily Amount, or RDA, for each. The RDA refers to the recommended level of intake for nutrients as determined by the United Kingdom Department of Health and Social Security (DHSS).

◆ Calcium deficiency may result in osteoporosis, or bone shrinking and weakening, in the elderly. Among those most at risk from this disease are women who repeatedly adopt low-calorie, low-fat diets that lack many of the best calcium sources. Calcium deficiency is also linked with periodontal disease and may contribute to high blood pressure. Two of the best sources of calcium are semi-skimmed and skimmed milk. However, milk products are not the only source of calcium, as the box opposite shows.

◆ Iron is vital to oxygen transport within the body. Women who exercise strenuously and who diet are particularly at risk from iron deficiency. If you reduce your intake of red meat, the best natural source of dietary iron, try to eat some of the foods listed on the opposite page. The iron in vegetables, fruits, grains and beans can be better absorbed by the body when these foods are eaten with small amounts of animal protein and foods that contain vitamin C (such as citrus fruits or tomatoes).

◆ Niacin and thiamine may be a problem for those on weight-loss diets, since these two B vitamins are present mainly in fatty foods such as meat and nuts. Both vitamins play a vital role in releasing energy from the food you eat and in regulating brain and nerve function.

◆ Most adults should restrict sodium intake to 1,000 milligrams per 1,000 calories consumed. One way to keep sodium consumption in check is to avoid adding table salt to food.

F O U R K E Y N U T R I E N T S

The foods listed below are good sources of the important vitamins and minerals covered in the guidelines on the opposite page. Many of them are included in the recipes in this book and may already be part of your diet. If they are not, incorporating them in your meals will help ensure adequate nutrition.

CALCIUM	mg	calories
RDA: Women 500 mg; men 500 mg		
Sardines, canned, with bones, 90 grams	371	175
Low-fat yogurt, 15 centilitres	270	78
Skimmed milk, 20 centilitres	247	63
Cheddar cheese, 30 grams	226	115
Tofu, 100 grams	159-507*	70
Broccoli tops, cooked, 100 grams	100	23
Spring greens, cooked, 100 grams	86	10
Molasses, blackstrap, 1 tablespoon	75	39
Cottage cheese, low-fat (4%), 100 grams	60	96

Even if you cut down on some dairy products to reduce fat intake, you can still get a good supply of calcium from low-fat dairy products and green vegetables.

IRON	mg	calories
RDA: Women 12 mg; men 10 mg		
Vitamin-mineral fortified cereal, 30 grams	18.0	100
Liver, lamb's, braised, 90 grams	8.0	152
Potato, baked, with skin, 200 grams	2.7	216
Haricot beans, cooked, 100 grams	2.5	93
Prawns, raw, 100 grams	1.8	117
Apricots, dried, 10 halves	1.7	83
Broccoli tops, cooked, 100 grams	1.5	23
Molasses, blackstrap, 1 tablespoon	1.4	39

Liver, one of the best iron sources, should not be eaten often because it is high in fat and cholesterol. The other foods listed are low in fat and most have no cholesterol.

THIAMINE	mg	calories
RDA: Women 0.9 mg; men 1.1 mg		
Brewer's yeast, 1 tablespoon	1.25	25
Pork, lean leg, roast, 90 grams	0.72	157
Fortified branflakes cereal, 30 grams	0.28	85
Peas, cooked, 100 grams	0.25	52
Peanuts, raw, 30 grams	0.25	160
Oatmeal, 30 grams	0.14	113
Asparagus, cooked, 100 grams	0.1	18

Thiamine, a B vitamin, must be constantly replenished because the body does not store it effectively. Fortified cereals, whole grains and pulses are low-fat sources.

NIACIN	mg	calories
RDA: Women 15 mg; men 18 mg		
Tuna, water-packed, 90 grams	10.0	95
Chicken breast, skinless, roast, 90 grams	8.7	139
Rump steak, lean only, grilled, 90 grams	6.3	168
Halibut, steamed, 100 grams	5.0	131
Oysters, 100 grams	1.5	51
Red kidney beans, cooked, 100 grams	0.5	128

Peanut butter, one of the best niacin sources, is high in fat. Lean meat, poultry, fish, shellfish and pulses are lower in fat and provide good amounts of niacin.

*Higher calcium figures are due to calcium added during processing

Keeping Track

Studies of people who change their eating habits show that keeping a diary is an important tool for successful weight control. Immediately writing down what you eat whenever you eat ensures your awareness of your food intake. Likewise, keeping a record of the exercise that you do demonstrates how active you are.

When examined at the end of a week or more, the daily eating and exercise diary provides an accurate picture of your behaviour patterns as well. You can compile your own diary by photocopying the opposite page, or you can create your own.

Start your diary at least one week before you plan to change your eating and exercise habits. During that first week, eat and exercise as usual. Do not eliminate any high-calorie foods that you ordinarily consume, and do not indulge in overly large portions of fattening dishes as a last indulgence before you begin cutting calories. Also, stick to your normal exercise regimen. Your diary for this period should give an accurate picture of your typical meals, snacks and activities. When you compare your normal pattern to your new habits, you can begin to assess their impact on your weight.

In the diet section of your diary, together with the foods you consume, make a note of where you eat, the distractions that are present and the mood you are in. All these observations are aids for identifying and then changing habitual patterns that contribute to overeating.

After a week, examine your diary for habits that contribute to your excess weight. Note the times and places that you are most likely to eat fattening snack foods.

Another important item worth analysing is what other activities you perform while you eat. Eating on the move or in your car and nibbling while you are preparing a meal are common habits to avoid when you are cutting calories from your diet.

If you find that you cannot resist buying high-fat snacks in the supermarket, you can schedule your shopping trips for after a meal, when you feel full. Or, if you find that you eat to offset depression at a certain hour of the day or day of the week, you can plan another kind of mood-elevating activity, such as exercise, for that period.

Then, after you have begun a low-calorie diet, use your diary to chart your progress. Are there problem areas in your daily diet that are particularly hard to change? Instead of abstaining from snacks at work, for example, try substituting low-calorie foods such as raw vegetables. You will probably find that switching to alternative foods is far easier than eliminating the habit entirely.

An advantage of keeping a diary while you are cutting calories is that the very act of writing down what you eat may act as a deterrent to overeating. You may be better able to resist a tempting, fattening food if you know your diary will act as a silent witness.

Once you reach your desired weight, continue your diary for a few weeks to make sure that you retain your new eating habits. At this stage of your weight programme, the diary will act as a reinforcement of your newly acquired habits.

Daily Eating and Exercise Diary

DATE

TIME	FOOD	AMOUNT	PLACE	DISTRACTIONS	MOOD

EXERCISE	TIME	PLACE	DURATION	MOOD

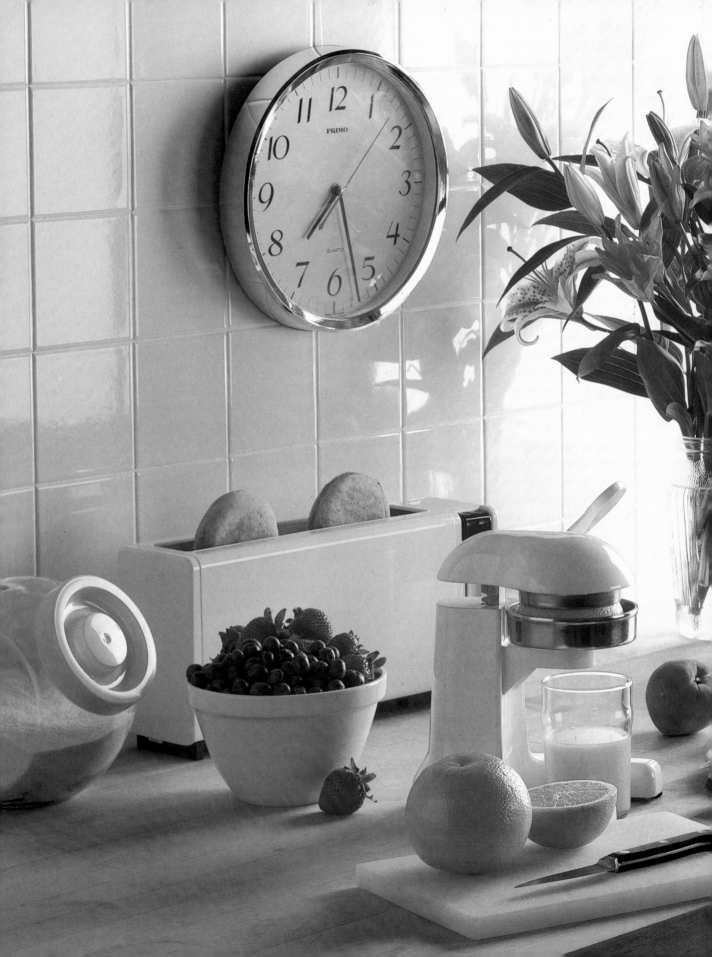

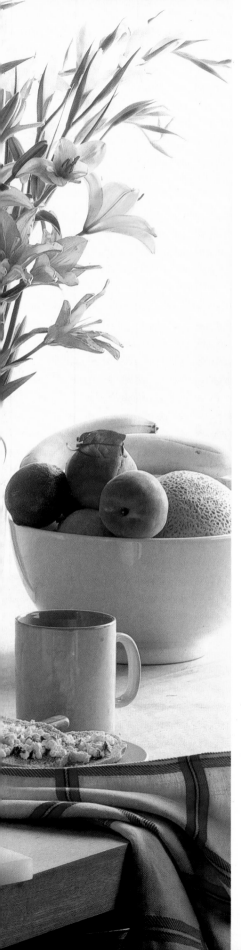

Breakfast

A filling start to the day

If you are trying to lose weight, you may be skimping on breakfast or missing it altogether. Either out of concern for their weight or because they are rushed in the morning, millions of people — one out of every four adults — forego breakfast most or all of the time. And surveys show that breakfast is more likely to be skipped than lunch or dinner. In fact, there is no evidence to suggest that skipping breakfast helps produce weight loss; indeed, a case can be made that eating early in the day is one of the best steps you can take towards achieving that goal.

As a means of controlling calories, the chief advantage of starting the day with a good breakfast is that it helps keep you from overeating later. A national food-consumption survey in the United States found that those who did not breakfast were more likely to resort to snacks later and to consume snacks higher in calories than breakfast eaters.

The person who eats little or no breakfast may eat an unusually large lunch, or else skimp on lunch, nibble throughout the afternoon and then eat a great deal at dinner. Yet for people concerned about their weight, evening may not be the best time to consume the bulk of their calories. In several recent studies, two groups of subjects were fed once a day, either at breakfast or at dinner. Both groups consumed the same number of calories. Most of the subjects on the morning-meal regimen lost more weight than those who ate in the evening. Although the studies involved only a handful of subjects, the research suggests that the body may burn calories eaten in the morning more readily than those eaten at night.

Of course, what you eat for this meal is as important as whether you eat it. Some traditional breakfast foods, such as eggs, bacon, sausage, cream, butter and whole milk are very high in fat and cholesterol. Even a modest breakfast comprising these foods can add up to 800 calories. An increasingly popular form of breakfast — the breakfast sandwich served in fast-food restaurants — is likewise high in calories and fat: in a survey of fast-food breakfast dishes, several of the sandwiches containing eggs and meat had more than 500 calories each, with 60 per cent or more of the calories coming from fat.

A breakfast consisting mainly of high-fat foods not only inhibits weight loss, but is also nutritionally unsound: the saturated fat in eggs, meat and dairy products tends to raise cholesterol levels, and fatty foods are generally low in the vitamins and minerals, particularly vitamin C and calcium, which make up a healthy diet. Skipping breakfast avoids fat, but it also deprives you of nutrients. Nor is your body properly fuelled on a meal of coffee and toast.

There are many strategies you can adopt to make breakfasts that are nourishing and also help you control your weight. First, you can choose low-fat versions of traditional breakfast foods. For example, instead of whole milk, which has 150 calories per 20 centilitre glass, use skimmed milk, which has only 63. Use egg whites rather than whole eggs: all the fat and cholesterol are in the yolk. Egg whites are an excellent source of protein and they help bind ingredients, as in the Gingerbread-Brown Rice Griddle Cakes on page 64. An alternative to butter is low-fat cheese, such as the ricotta used on the Cornmeal-Cheese Muffins on page 54. You can avoid excessive sugar at breakfast by trying home-made fruit juices and sauces, which make nutritious low-calorie sweeteners — for example, as a topping for the French Toast Fingers on page 50.

Second, expand your definition of what is suitable as a breakfast dish. There is no reason why vegetables and pulses, which are relatively low in calories and high in fibre and complex carbohydrates, cannot be eaten in the morning — and these foods have the benefit of filling you up, as do less familiar whole grains such as burghul. A wide variety of foods are explored in many of the recipes that follow, such as the Oatmeal-Burghul Cereal with Tangerines on page 51, Tortillas Rancheras, filled with vegetables and beans, on page 52 and Baked Sweet Potato Doughnuts on page 56.

▼ Most of the main-dish recipes in this chapter have from 300 to 395 calories per serving. Certain recipes, marked with a triangle, are extra-low in calories — between 100 and 250 per serving. These can be eaten alone, or they can be combined with other foods. The mid-morning snacks in the section following main dishes all have fewer than 200 calories.

Choosing a Cereal

Ready-to-eat cereals are not only convenient, but can offer a filling low-calorie breakfast. Studies show that people who eat cereal for breakfast generally consume less fat and fewer calories than those who rely on other conventional breakfast foods. Unfortunately, some popular cereals are loaded with refined sugar and fat. The following suggestions will help you choose a packaged cereal that gives you the most nutritive value for your calories.

◆ Study the cereal box label. In general, the shorter the list of ingredients, the more nutritious the cereal. Ideally, a whole grain should be listed first: this means it is the main component. Thirty grams of cereal, the amount usually given as one serving, can range from 50 to 130 calories. Most of these calories are from carbohydrates, but be sure that they are from the complex variety — grains — rather than from simple sugars. In some popular cereals, refined sweeteners make up 40 to 60 per cent of the weight, the equivalent of four heaped teaspoons of sugar in 30 grams of cereal. The ratio (in grams) of total carbohydrates to protein should be about 8 to 1. If the ratio is greater, the cereal probably provides too much refined sugar.

◆ Most ready-to-eat cereals are relatively low in fat, with one to three grams per 30 gram serving. But granola cereals tend to have much more fat than other types — at least four grams per 30 gram serving, as much as a pat and a half of butter. Most of this fat may be highly saturated palm oil or coconut oil, both of which can contribute to raised cholesterol levels. You are better off eating home-made granola, prepared with as little oil as possible.

◆ Cereals can be a good source of dietary fibre, which is one of the best food components to help control weight *(pages 46-47)*.

Third, some advance planning can simplify your morning routine so that you have time to eat and enjoy breakfast. Bake breads or muffins in advance or, for recipes with short cooking times, measure out and prepare the ingredients the night before.

If you are one of those people who has no appetite until you have been up for an hour or two — and you have to be at work early — take something nourishing with you when you leave home in the morning. If you do eat a full breakfast but still get hungry before lunch, keep your hunger at bay with one of the light, nutritious snacks on pages 70-73. An essential component of a weight-loss regimen is for you to feel relatively full until it is time for your next meal. You can achieve that feeling with fewer calories than you might expect.

Finally, when you have no time or inclination to cook, you can put together a low-calorie quick breakfast. Quick Oats with Mixed Fruit on page 59 takes only minutes to make, as do the fruit milk shakes on pages 52 and 64. Ready-to-eat cereals with fruit and semi-skimmed milk also provide quick, satisfying meals as long as you keep sound nutrition in mind when choosing your cereal *(see box, above)*.

Feeling Full

There is no mystery as to why a traditional breakfast of eggs, bacon and buttered toast fills you up. Such a meal is high in fat, and fat slows up the process of food leaving your stomach, making you feel full. But you can achieve the same result without eating fatty foods. People who regularly consume foods high in dietary fibre find it easier to keep their weight down since fibre is filling but does not add calories.

Fibre is the part- of plants that passes through your system undigested after you have eaten them. The bran in whole-grain breads and cereals is probably the most familiar form of fibre, but — as indicated opposite — fruit, vegetables, oats, nuts and pulses such as kidney beans and lentils are also high-fibre foods.

One characteristic of cellulose, the fibre most commonly found in whole grains, is that it absorbs water, which helps contribute to a feeling of fullness. Fibre expands quickly in the stomach and small intestine so that you feel satisfied sooner, and the sensation of fullness lasts relatively long. The texture of high-fibre foods can also make them take longer to chew than foods high in fat, and this helps slow down your eating. Not only do fibrous foods have fewer calories than fatty foods, they also tend to be better sources of vitamin A and the mineral potassium.

Recent recommendations of the National Advisory Committee on Nutrition Education in the United Kingdom are that adults should consume 30 grams of dietary fibre daily. Most Britons consume only 16 to 20 grams daily. If you should increase your fibre intake, do so gradually; otherwise, you may irritate the lining of your intestines or suffer gas or bloating. Here are some suggestions for getting more fibre into your diet:

• Eat a variety of foods. This will help ensure that you get the benefits of various forms of fibre. By aiding the passage of food through the large intestine, insoluble fibres such as cellulose not only fill you up, but may also help prevent intestinal disorders, from constipation to colon cancer. Water-soluble fibres such as pectins, which are found mainly in fruits, vegetables, and grains such as barley and oats, do less to help the passage of food, but they appear to lower blood cholesterol.

• Eat raw fruits and vegetables as a mid-morning snack. Fruit and vegetables such as apples, carrots and broccoli are rich in fibre, but they should be eaten raw — boiling, peeling and processing tend to reduce the fibre content of these foods.

• Drink liquids when you eat high-fibre foods. Water and other fluids help you feel full by taking up space in your stomach. And when consumed with sufficient fluids, fibre helps regulate bowel function.

• Spread out your fibre intake. Breakfast is an excellent time to eat high-fibre foods, particularly cereals. Getting all your fibre at one sitting, however, may increase the chance of unpleasant side effects. As a rule, you should have foods containing fibre that is both water-soluble and water-insoluble at every meal.

HIGH-FIBRE FOODS

Food	Serving	Dietary Fibre (grams)
Haricot beans, cooked	100 grams	7.4
Kidney beans, cooked	100 grams	7.0
Spinach, cooked	100 grams	6.3
Pear with skin	1 large	6.2
Peas, cooked	100 grams	5.2
Puffed wheat	30 grams	4.6
Almonds	30 grams	4.2
Broccoli tops, cooked	100 grams	4.1
Raspberries	60 grams	4.1
Blackberries	60 grams	4.0
Turnips, cooked	100 grams	3.9
Spaghetti, wholemeal	100 grams	3.8
Lentils, cooked	100 grams	3.7
Apple with skin	1 medium	3.5
Muesli	30 grams	3.4
Sweet potato, cooked	1 medium	3.4
Wheat, shredded	30 grams	3.4
Carrots, cooked	100 grams	3.1
Cornflakes	30 grams	3.1
Prunes	3	3.0
French beans, cooked	100 grams	2.9
Brussels sprouts, cooked	100 grams	2.9
Orange	1 medium	2.6
Bread, wholemeal	1 large slice	2.5
Cabbage, cooked	100 grams	2.5
Parsnips, cooked	100 grams	2.5
Potato with skin, cooked	1 medium	2.5
Banana	1 medium	2.4
Dates	3	1.9
Peach with skin	1 medium	1.9
Raisins	30 grams	1.9
Celery, raw	60 grams	1.8
Asparagus, cooked	100 grams	1.5
Bean sprouts, raw	60 grams	1.5
Spaghetti, boiled	100 grams	1.5
Tomatoes, raw	100 grams	1.5
Apricots, dried	5 halves	1.4
Cherries	10	1.2
Pineapple	100 grams	1.2
Bread, white	30 grams	1.1
Brown rice, cooked	100 grams	1.1
Cantaloupe melon	100 grams	1.0
Lettuce, raw	60 grams	0.8

Continuous Callisthenics

A callisthenics routine at the start of the day provides an excellent non-stressful way to raise your metabolism and your body temperature. Callisthenics can also burn 100 to 200 calories or more in less than half an hour if it is performed vigorously.

The exercises on this and the opposite page are meant to follow one another as a continuous series. Perform each exercise for several minutes so that the routine adds up to a 20-minute workout.

Jogging on the spot is an excellent way to warm up and cool down, since you can easily regulate its intensity. Before you begin your routine, jog on the spot for three to five minutes, gradually increasing the intensity until you break into a light sweat. After you have completed the callisthenics routine, jog on the spot again for five minutes to serve as a cool-down.

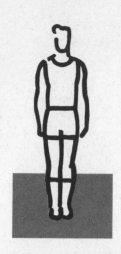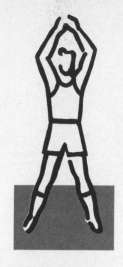

1. To perform jumping jacks, stand with your feet together and your hands at your sides. Jump so that your feet land apart and your hands touch above your head. Make sure that your heels touch the ground when you land. Return to the starting position and repeat.

2. Perform a series of heel touches. First, stand with your feet apart and your hands touching above your head. Squat down and touch your ankles. Return to the standing position and repeat. Do not bend your knees more than 90°.

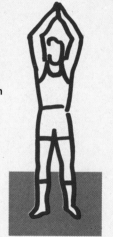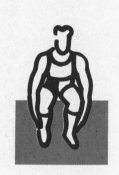

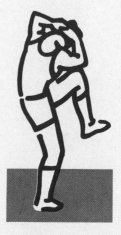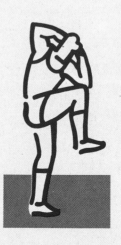

3. Interlace your fingers behind your head and lift your left knee to touch it with your right elbow. Alternate right knee and left elbow and back again.

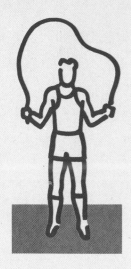

4. Skip with a two-footed bounce, landing on the balls of your feet with your knees slightly bent. Jump no more than a couple of centimetres in the air to avoid the risk of injury.

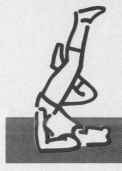

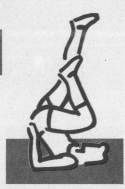

5. Lie on your back, lift your feet towards the ceiling and support your pelvis with your hands. Alternately kick up and down as if you were pedalling a bicycle. Avoid taking your body weight on the neck.

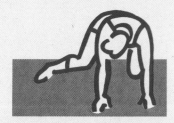

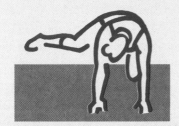

6. Kneel on all fours and extend one foot out to the side *(far left)*. Keep your knee slightly flexed and raise your leg. Then repeat for the opposite leg.

7. Perform hip and leg extensions by kneeling on all fours and drawing your right knee to your chin. Swing your right leg out and up, then bring it back to your chin. Swing one leg, then the other.

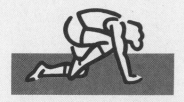

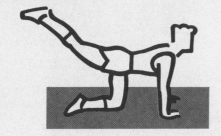

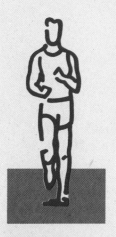

8. Run on the spot and gradually reduce your exercise intensity to cool down. Spend at least three to five minutes cooling down.

FRENCH TOAST FINGERS WITH APPLE PURÉE

A warm, unsweetened fruit sauce tops this wholemeal French toast.

CALORIES per serving	350
59% Carbohydrate	55 g
13% Protein	12 g
28% Fat	11 g
CALCIUM	92 mg
IRON	3 mg
SODIUM	318 mg

4 Granny Smith apples, peeled, cored and thinly sliced (about 550 g/1 lb 2 oz total weight)
25 cl (8 fl oz) apple juice
1 teaspoon lemon juice
Pinch of grated lemon rind
Pinch of mixed spice
100 g (3½ oz) sultanas

30 g (1 oz) shelled walnuts, chopped
3 large eggs, plus 4 egg whites
3 tablespoons skimmed milk
1 teaspoon pure vanilla extract
¼ teaspoon ground cinnamon
5 teaspoons vegetable oil
12 slices wholemeal bread

Cook the apples, apple juice, lemon juice, rind and mixed spice in a medium-sized pan over medium heat for 10 minutes; process in a food processor or blender until puréed but still chunky. Stir in the sultanas and walnuts, return the purée to the pan and cover to keep warm. In a large, shallow bowl whisk together the eggs, egg whites and milk. Add the vanilla and cinnamon. Heat 2 teaspoons of the oil in a large non-stick frying pan over medium-high heat. Dip four slices of bread into the egg mixture, place them in the pan and cook for 3 minutes. Turn and cook for another 3 minutes, or until well browned. Dip and cook the remaining bread in the same way, adding oil as necessary. Cut each piece of French toast into four strips, divide them among six plates and top each serving with the apple purée. Makes 6 servings

French Toast Fingers with Apple Purée

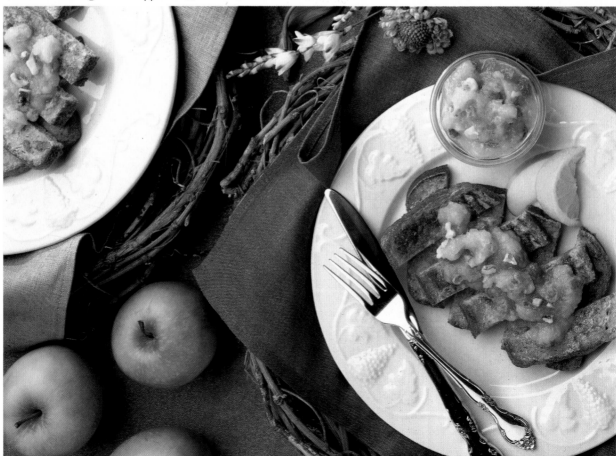

OATMEAL BURGHUL CEREAL WITH TANGERINES

Burghul and oats are good sources of iron, a mineral that is often lacking in low-calorie diets. Tangerines contribute vitamin C, which aids in the absorption of iron, and they also provide your daily vitamin A requirement.

CALORIES per serving	365
74% Carbohydrate	69 g
15% Protein	14 g
11% Fat	4 g
CALCIUM	195 mg
IRON	3 mg
SODIUM	98 mg

125 g (4 oz) burghul
160 g (5½ oz) rolled oats
Pinch of salt
¼ teaspoon ground cinnamon

50 cl (16 fl oz) semi-skimmed milk
4 tangerines, peeled and
  segmented
1 teaspoon grated lime rind

Place the burghul in a medium-sized bowl, add 25 cl (8 fl oz) of hot water and set aside for about 20 minutes, or until the burghul is slightly softened.

Place the oats in a medium-sized saucepan and add the salt, burghul and 1 litre (1¾ pints) of water. Bring to the boil over medium heat and cook for 5 minutes, then reduce the heat to low and simmer for another 3 minutes, or until the cereal is thickened. Stir in the cinnamon, then spoon the cereal into four bowls and pour some of the milk over each serving. Top with the tangerine segments, sprinkle with the lime rind and serve.   Makes 4 servings

WHOLE-GRAIN SODA BREAD

The whole grains in this bread provide insoluble fibre, which may help prevent some types of cancer, and the oats, nuts and raisins contain a type of fibre that has been shown to lower elevated blood cholesterol levels. High-fibre breads keep you feeling full longer than refined flour products do.

CALORIES per serving	335
70% Carbohydrate	62 g
10% Protein	9 g
20% Fat	8 g
CALCIUM	164 mg
IRON	3 mg
SODIUM	434 mg

4 tablespoons wheat berries
  (whole-wheat grains)
125 g (4 oz) raisins
125 g (4 oz) wholemeal flour
75 g (2½ oz) plain flour
45 g (1½ oz) rolled oats
30 g (1 oz) shelled walnuts,
  chopped
45 g (1½ oz) dark brown sugar

2 teaspoons caraway seeds
2 teaspoons baking powder
1 teaspoon bicarbonate of soda
¼ teaspoon salt
25 cl (8 fl oz) plus 2 teaspoons
  buttermilk
1 large egg
1 tablespoon vegetable oil
4 tablespoons honey

Place the wheat berries in a small bowl, add 12.5 cl (4 fl oz) of boiling water and set aside to soak for 1 hour, or until soft. Place the raisins in another small bowl, add hot water to cover and set aside to soak.

Preheat the oven to 190°C (375°F or Mark 5). Lightly oil a 22 cm (9 inch) round baking tin; set aside. Drain the wheat berries and raisins. In a large bowl, stir together the wholemeal flour, plain flour, oats, walnuts, sugar, caraway seeds, baking powder, bicarbonate of soda and salt; make a well in the centre. Pour in 25 cl (8 fl oz) of the buttermilk, the egg and oil and stir to blend. Add the drained wheat berries and raisins and stir just until the mixture forms a soft dough; do not overmix. Spoon the dough into the prepared tin, mounding it slightly in the centre, and brush it with the remaining buttermilk. Bake the bread in the centre of the oven for 35 to 40 minutes, or until the loaf is golden-brown and sounds hollow when removed from the pan and tapped on the bottom. Transfer the loaf to a wire rack to cool for 10 minutes, then cut it into 12 wedges and serve with the honey.   Makes 6 servings

TORTILLAS RANCHERAS

Vegetables and beans make this Tex-Mex dish a fibre-rich brunch.

CALORIES per serving	315
59% Carbohydrate	48 g
17% Protein	14 g
24% Fat	9 g
CALCIUM	125 mg
IRON	6 mg
SODIUM	20 mg

350 g (12 oz) diced tomatoes
150 g (5 oz) sweet yellow pepper, diced
150 g (5 oz) sweet red pepper, diced
45 g (1½ oz) spring onions, finely chopped
4 tablespoons chopped fresh coriander
4 tablespoons fresh lime juice
Pinch of grated lime rind

½ teaspoon chili powder
½ teaspoon ground cumin
Pinch of hot red pepper flakes
275 g (9 oz) cooked black beans (135 g/4½ oz dried weight)
2 teaspoons vegetable oil
4 flour tortillas (recipe follows)
175 g (6 oz) cos lettuce, shredded
45 g (1½ oz) unsalted roasted peanuts

In a medium-sized bowl, stir together the tomatoes, sweet peppers, spring onions, coriander, lime juice, lime rind, chili powder, cumin and pepper flakes. Add the black beans and stir to combine; set aside.

Heat ½ teaspoon of the oil in a medium-sized non-stick frying pan over medium-high heat. Place a tortilla in the pan and cook for about 1 minute on each side, or until it is warmed and softened. Repeat with the remaining tortillas and place them on four plates. Top each tortilla with the shredded lettuce and the tomato mixture and sprinkle with the peanuts.   Makes 4 servings

FLOUR TORTILLAS

CALORIES per serving	150
46% Carbohydrate	18 g
8% Protein	3 g
46% Fat	8 g
CALCIUM	35 mg
IRON	Trace
SODIUM	65 mg

150 g (5 oz) plain flour
⅓ teaspoon salt

45 g (1½ oz) white vegetable fat

Mix the flour with the salt and rub in the fat. Gradually add 4½ tablespoons of warm water and knead the dough for 3 minutes. Put the dough in a bowl, cover it with plastic film and leave it to rest at room temperature for 15 minutes. Divide the dough into six equal pieces and roll each piece out on a floured board to make a 20 cm (8 inch) circle.

Cook each tortilla in a lightly greased non-stick frying pan or crêpe pan until bubbles form and the surface is lightly speckled — about 30 seconds. Using a wooden spoon or spatula, flatten the bubbles, then turn the tortilla over and cook it for 30 seconds on the other side.   Makes 6 tortillas

STRAWBERRY-ORANGE MILK SHAKE ▼

No sugar is added to this breakfast drink. It gets its sweetness — and its abundance of vitamin C and the mineral potassium — from fresh fruit.

CALORIES per serving	125
81% Carbohydrate	26 g
11% Protein	4 g
8% Fat	1 g
CALCIUM	97 mg
IRON	1 mg
SODIUM	67 mg

250 g (8 oz) strawberries, sliced
25 cl (8 fl oz) orange juice

½ small banana
12.5 cl (4 fl oz) buttermilk

Combine all the ingredients in a blender and process until smoothly blended. Pour the mixture into two tall glasses and serve.   Makes 2 servings

Tortillas Rancheras ▷

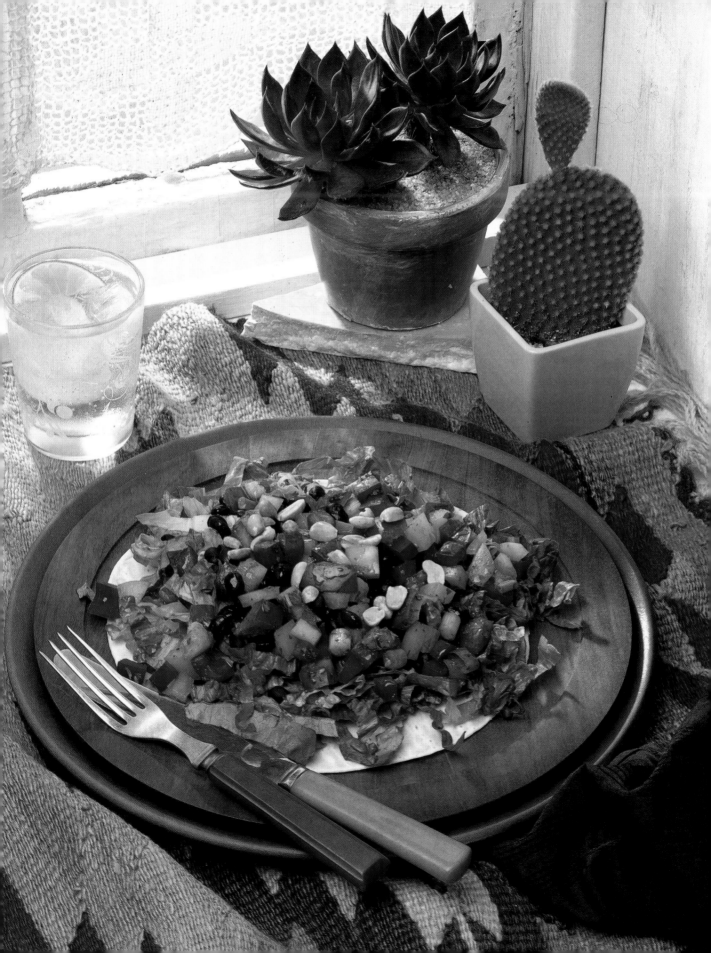

CORNMEAL-CHEESE MUFFINS

The ricotta topping served with these muffins is a good low-fat source of calcium. In contrast, butter derives 100 per cent of its calories from fat and provides no significant nutrients apart from vitamin A.

CALORIES per serving	335
69% Carbohydrate	64 g
14% Protein	13 g
17% Fat	5 g
CALCIUM	126 mg
IRON	3 mg
SODIUM	444 mg

175 g (6 oz) frozen sweetcorn
  kernels
175 g (6 oz) plain flour,
  approximately
125 g (4 oz) cornmeal,
  approximately
125 g (4 oz) wholemeal flour
¾ teaspoon salt
¾ teaspoon pepper

30 g (1 oz) blue cheese, crumbled
1 large egg white
2 teaspoons vegetable oil
7 g (¼ oz) dried yeast
½ tablespoon honey
125 g (4 oz) low-fat ricotta cheese
2 tablespoons finely chopped
  spring onions

Place the sweetcorn in a food processor and process for about 10 seconds, or until chopped. Remove about half of the sweetcorn and set aside. Add the plain flour, cornmeal, wholemeal flour, salt, pepper, blue cheese, egg white and oil to the food processor and cover it; set aside. Place the yeast in a small cup, add 4 tablespoons of warm water (40-45°C/105-115°F) and the honey and set aside for about 5 minutes, or until foamy.

Stir the yeast mixture. Start the food processor, pour in the yeast mixture through the feed tube and process for about 40 seconds. Add the reserved sweetcorn and process for another 5 seconds; the dough should form a ball. Place the dough in a medium-sized bowl, cover it with a tea towel and set aside in a warm place to rise for 1 hour, or until the dough is doubled in bulk.

Sprinkle a baking sheet with 2 teaspoons of cornmeal. Knock back the dough and on a lightly floured board roll it out to an 8 mm (⅜ inch) thickness. Using an 9 cm (3½ inch) cutter, cut out six muffins. Transfer the muffins to the baking sheet, cover with a tea towel and set aside in a warm place to rise for 25 minutes, or until the muffins are about 1½ times their original size.

Heat a medium-sized non-stick frying pan over medium heat. Using a metal spatula place three muffins in the pan and cook for about 6 minutes, or until the bottoms of the muffins are golden-brown. Turn the muffins and cook for another 6 minutes. Transfer the cooked muffins to a wire rack to cool and cook the remaining muffins in the same way.

Just before serving, stir together the ricotta and spring onions in a small bowl. Split and toast the muffins, then spread each half with 2 teaspoons of the ricotta spread and serve. Makes 6 servings

Note: the muffins can be made in advance and frozen, but the spread should only be made shortly before serving, or the flavour of the spring onions may become unpleasantly strong.

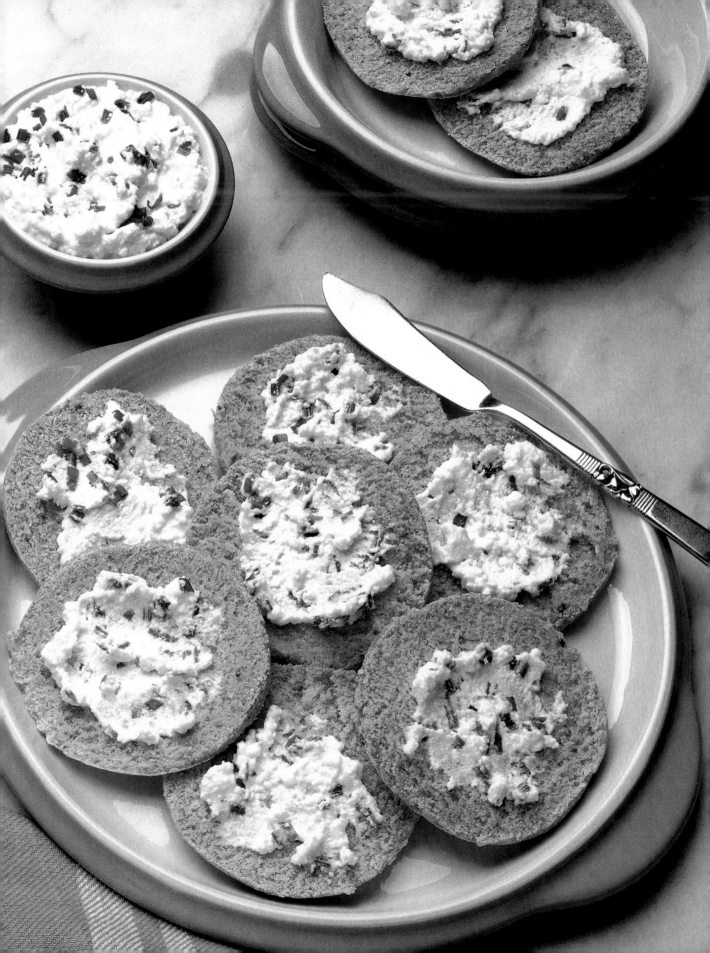

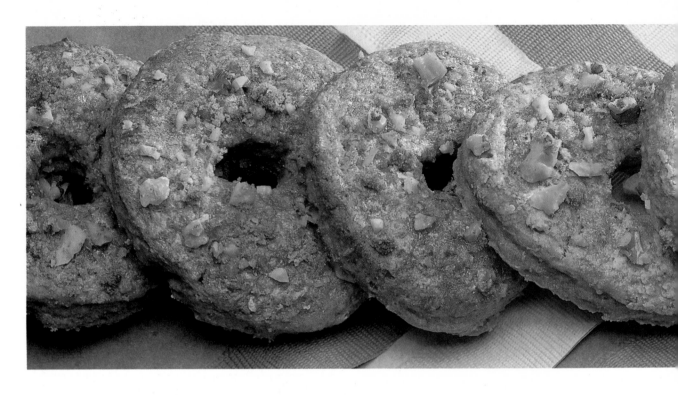

BAKED SWEET POTATO DOUGHNUTS

These doughnuts are filling because of their high fibre content. And because they are baked rather than deep fried, they are far more healthy than ordinary doughnuts.

CALORIES per serving	275
66% Carbohydrate	46 g
9% Protein	7 g
25% Fat	8 g
CALCIUM	109 mg
IRON	2 mg
SODIUM	329 mg

1 orange-fleshed sweet potato (about 175 g/6 oz)
150 g (5 oz) plain flour, approximately
90 g (3 oz) wholemeal flour
2 teaspoons baking powder
½ teaspoon bicarbonate of soda
1 teaspoon ground cinnamon
¼ teaspoon grated nutmeg

¼ teaspoon salt
1 large egg, plus 1 egg white
2 tablespoons vegetable oil
5 tablespoons light brown sugar
2 tablespoons apple juice concentrate
2 tablespoons chopped shelled walnuts

Place the sweet potato in a small saucepan with cold water to cover and bring to the boil over medium-high heat. Cook the potato for about 35 minutes, or until fork-tender; drain. When the sweet potato is cool enough to handle, peel it, place it in a large bowl and mash it; set aside.

Preheat the oven to 220°C (425°F or Mark 7). In a small bowl, stir together the flours, baking powder, bicarbonate of soda, spices and salt; set aside. In another small bowl, beat the egg white with a fork, then add 1 tablespoon to the mashed potato. Reserve the remaining egg white. Add the whole egg, oil, 4 tablespoons of the sugar and the apple juice concentrate to the potato and mix well. Add the dry ingredients and stir to form a dough.

Lightly oil a baking sheet; set aside. Turn the dough out on to a lightly floured board, knead it a few times and roll it out to an 8 mm (⅜ inch) thickness. Using a 7.5 cm (3 inch) doughnut cutter, cut out six doughnuts. Mix the

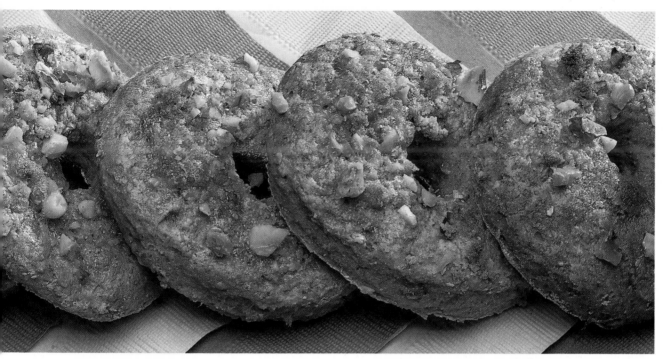

walnuts and remaining sugar on a small plate. (For less sweet doughnuts, omit the sugar from the topping.) Brush the tops and cut-out centres of the doughnuts with the remaining egg white, dip them in the walnut topping and place them on the baking sheet. Bake the doughnuts for 13 to 15 minutes, or until the tops are golden and the bottoms are lightly browned. Transfer to a rack to cool briefly, and serve warm.   Makes 6 servings

FRUIT WITH LEMON YOGURT SAUCE

Each generous serving of this fresh fruit salad provides more than half of the calcium, one third of the phosphorus and all the vitamins A and C you need daily; in addition it supplies a good amount of potassium.

CALORIES per serving	355
60% Carbohydrate	58 g
11% Protein	11 g
29% Fat	12 g
CALCIUM	272 mg
IRON	2 mg
SODIUM	100 mg

25 cl (8 fl oz) plain low-fat yogurt
1 tablespoon granulated sugar
2 teaspoons lemon juice
1½ teaspoons grated lemon rind
175 g (6 oz) cantaloupe melon
   flesh, diced
175 g (6 oz) honeydew melon
   flesh, diced
150 g (5 oz) fresh pineapple, diced

250 g (8 oz) fresh strawberries,
   sliced
60 g (2 oz) fresh raspberries
75 g (2½ oz) seedless red
   grapes
75 g (2½ oz) papaya flesh, diced
30 g (1 oz) shelled walnuts,
   chopped

For the sauce, stir together the yogurt, sugar, lemon juice and lemon rind in a small bowl; set aside. Place all the fruit in a large bowl and toss gently to combine. Divide the fruit mixture between two bowls, top each serving with half of the sauce and sprinkle with the walnuts.   Makes 2 servings

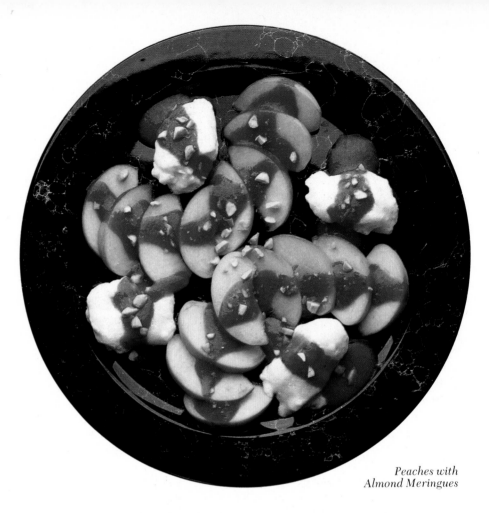

*Peaches with
Almond Meringues*

PEACHES WITH ALMOND MERINGUES ▼

CALORIES per serving	200
70% Carbohydrate	38 g
12% Protein	6 g
18% Fat	4 g
CALCIUM	35 mg
IRON	1 mg
SODIUM	51 mg

*For low-calorie cooking, try to use more egg whites than yolks: a large egg
white has 3 grams of protein, no fat and no cholesterol, whereas the yolk
has nearly 6 grams of fat and about 275 milligrams of cholesterol.*

4 purple plums, halved and
  stoned
Pinch of cinnamon
4 peaches, halved and stoned

4 egg whites, at room temperature
4 tablespoons caster sugar
12 toasted blanched almonds,
  chopped

For the sauce, coarsely chop the plums. Process them in a food processor or
blender with the cinnamon for 1 minute, or until smooth. Sieve the sauce; set
aside. Cut the peaches into 1 cm (½ inch) thick slices; set aside.

For the meringues, fill a large frying pan three-quarters full of water and
bring it to a simmer over medium heat. Meanwhile, in a large bowl, beat the
egg whites using an electric mixer until firm but not dry. Whisk in the sugar 1
tablespoon at a time, then whisk the egg whites for about 30 seconds, or until
glossy. Carefully place eight separate tablespoons of meringue in the simmering water and poach them for about 10 seconds, then flip them over and
poach for about 5 seconds, or just until firm. Using a slotted spoon, transfer
the meringues to a plate. Make another eight meringues in the same way. Arrange the peach slices and the meringues on four plates, spoon some plum
sauce over each serving and sprinkle with the almonds.　　　Makes 4 servings

CORN AND POTATO HASH

The vegetables in this dish provide plenty of fibre — 6 grams per serving, which is one fifth of the Recommended Daily Amount.

CALORIES per serving	290
56% Carbohydrate	45 g
15% Protein	10 g
29% Fat	11 g
CALCIUM	37 mg
IRON	2 mg
SODIUM	435 mg

500 g (1 lb) potatoes, peeled and coarsely diced
250 g (8 oz) fresh or frozen sweetcorn kernels
2 tablespoons olive oil
1 large sweet green pepper, coarsely diced

2 onions, coarsely diced
90 g (3 oz) lean back bacon, diced
2 teaspoons cumin seeds
½ teaspoon black pepper
Tabasco sauce to taste
2 tomatoes, coarsely diced
4 spring onions, thinly sliced

Bring a medium-sized saucepan of water to the boil over medium-high heat, add the potatoes and cook for 10 minutes, or until soft. Meanwhile, cook the sweetcorn in boiling water for 3 to 4 minutes or until tender. Drain both the potatoes and the corn well. In a large bowl, mash the potatoes lightly with a fork and mix in the sweetcorn. Set aside. Heat 2 teaspoons of the oil in a saucepan over medium-high heat. Add the pepper, onions and bacon and cook, stirring, for 3 minutes or until the vegetables begin to wilt. Add 2 tablespoons of water, cover, reduce the heat to low and cook for 10 minutes, or until the vegetables are soft. Meanwhile, toast the cumin seeds in a small dry frying pan over high heat, shaking the seeds in the pan for 1 minute, or until they are fragrant and brown. Crush the seeds in a mortar with a pestle. Add the cumin to the potatoes and sweetcorn together with the cooked pepper, onion and bacon, black pepper and some Tabasco sauce; mix well.

Heat 1 tablespoon of the remaining oil in a large frying pan, then add the potato mixture, pressing it into a large, flat, round cake in the pan. Cook over medium-high heat for 3 to 4 minutes or until golden-brown underneath. Place a large plate on top of the pan, then invert both the plate and pan together so that the potato cake is turned out on to the plate. Heat the remaining oil in the pan, then carefully slide the potato cake back into the pan. Cook the other side for 3 to 4 minutes, until golden-brown. Sprinkle the tomatoes and spring onions over the potato cake. Serve from the pan.   Makes 4 servings

QUICK OATS WITH MIXED FRUIT

Quick-cooking oats have the same amount of cholesterol-lowering oat bran as old-fashioned porridge oats — in fact, the two are nutritionally identical.

CALORIES per serving	300
84% Carbohydrate	67 g
10% Protein	8 g
6% Fat	2 g
CALCIUM	33 mg
IRON	2 mg
SODIUM	118 mg

17.5 cl (6 fl oz) apple juice
60 g (2 oz) quick-cooking porridge oats
Pinch of salt
Pinch of ground cinnamon

60 g (2 oz) mixed dried fruit, finely chopped
2 tablespoons honey
15 cl (¼ pint) skimmed milk

In a small saucepan, stir together the apple juice, oats, salt, cinnamon and 17.5 cl (6 fl oz) of water and bring to the boil over medium-high heat. Reduce the heat to low, cover the pan and simmer for 1 minute, or until the liquid is absorbed; remove from the heat. Stir in the fruit and honey, cover the pan and allow to stand for 2 minutes, or until the fruit is soft. Place the porridge in two bowls and pour half the milk over each serving.   Makes 2 servings

FRUIT AND RICE FRITTERS ▼

These healthy fritters are cooked in a fraction of the oil needed for deep frying. The dried fruit and brown rice supply fibre and minerals, notably iron and potassium.

CALORIES per serving	220
65% Carbohydrate	38 g
9% Protein	5 g
26% Fat	7 g
CALCIUM	28 mg
IRON	2 mg
SODIUM	121 mg

5 dried pear halves
5 dried peach halves
5 dried apricots
4 tablespoons wholemeal flour
225 g (7½ oz) cooked brown rice (90 g/3 oz raw)

1 large egg, separated, plus 2 egg whites
1 tablespoon toasted sesame seeds
¼ teaspoon salt
¼ teaspoon mixed spice
2 tablespoons vegetable oil

Finely chop the dried fruit, place it in a medium-sized bowl with the flour and toss to coat the fruit. Add the rice, egg yolk, sesame seeds, salt and mixed spice and mix well; set aside. In a large bowl, beat the egg whites until stiff, using an electric mixer. Gently fold the egg whites into the rice mixture. Heat the oil in a large non-stick frying pan over medium heat. Using 12.5 cl (4 fl oz) of batter for each, make three fritters, flattening them with a spatula to a 1 cm (½ inch) thickness. Cook for 2 to 3 minutes, then turn and cook for another 2 to 3 minutes, or until the fritters are golden on both sides. Make three more fritters in the same fashion and serve immediately. Makes 6 servings

BREAKFAST INDIAN PUDDINGS

Dark molasses is a source of calcium — the combination of molasses, milk and yogurt here provides about two thirds of the daily requirement.

CALORIES per serving	330
70% Carbohydrate	58 g
14% Protein	11 g
16% Fat	6 g
CALCIUM	380 mg
IRON	6 mg
SODIUM	172 mg

90 g (3 oz) cornmeal
4 tablespoons dark molasses
2 large eggs
1½ teaspoons ground cinnamon
1 teaspoon ground ginger
½ teaspoon grated nutmeg
Pinch of salt

50 cl (16 fl oz) semi-skimmed milk
25 cl (8 fl oz) apricot nectar
1 teaspoon pure vanilla extract
8 dried apricots
12.5 cl (4 fl oz) plain low-fat yogurt

Preheat the oven to 170°C (325°F or Mark 3). In a large bowl, whisk together the cornmeal, molasses, eggs, 1¼ teaspoons of the cinnamon, the ginger, nutmeg and salt; set aside. Heat the milk, apricot nectar and vanilla extract in a medium-sized pan over medium-high heat until hot. Whisk quarter of the hot liquid into the cornmeal mixture, then whisk in the remaining liquid. Return the mixture to the saucepan and cook, whisking constantly, for 2 minutes, or until it thickens and starts to bubble. Divide the mixture among four 25 cl (8 fl oz) ramekins and bake for about 40 minutes, or until firm and browned on top.

Let the puddings cool at room temperature for about 30 minutes. (If making them the night before, cover and refrigerate them when cool; reheat them in a 180°C/350°F or Mark 4 oven for 20 minutes.) A few minutes before serving, place the apricots in a small bowl and add boiling water to cover; allow to stand for 1 minute. Drain the apricots and cut them into strips. Top each pudding with 2 tablespoons of the yogurt and some apricot strips and sprinkle with the remaining cinnamon. Makes 4 servings

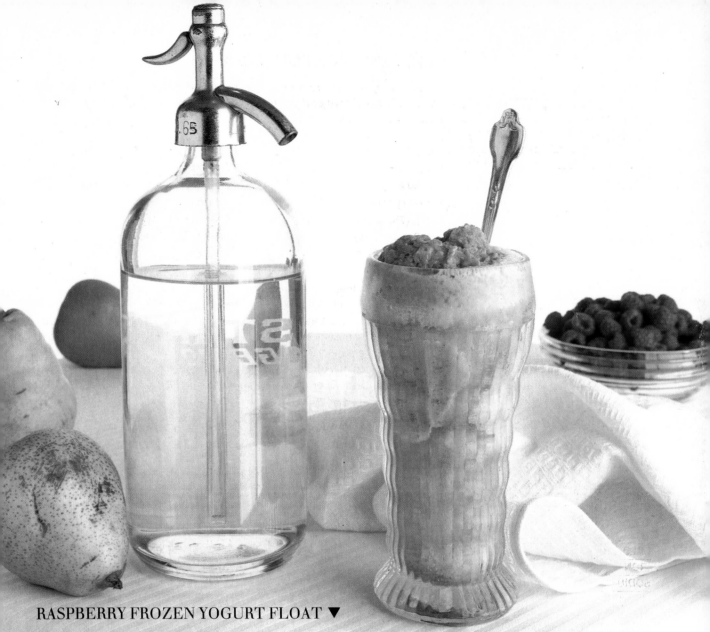

RASPBERRY FROZEN YOGURT FLOAT ▼

The frozen yogurt in this fibre and potassium-rich float can also be served
as a nutritious snack or dessert.

4 pears
250 g (8 oz) fresh or frozen
   raspberries
1 tablespoon pure maple syrup

75 cl (1¼ pints) plain low-fat
   yogurt
1 egg white
1 litre (1¾ pints) soda water

CALORIES per serving	170
65% Carbohydrate	30 g
25% Protein	11 g
10% Fat	8 g
CALCIUM	373 mg
IRON	1 mg
SODIUM	171 mg

Peel, core and dice the pears. Purée the raspberries in a food processor or
blender; sieve the purée into a small bowl and set aside. Purée the pears,
then add the raspberry purée, the maple syrup, yogurt, and egg white, and
process until thoroughly combined. Transfer the mixture to a shallow metal
container, cover with plastic film and place in the freezer overnight.

Thaw the frozen yogurt at room temperature for 30 minutes, or until slightly
soft. Scoop into four tall glasses, top up with soda water and serve.

Makes 4 servings

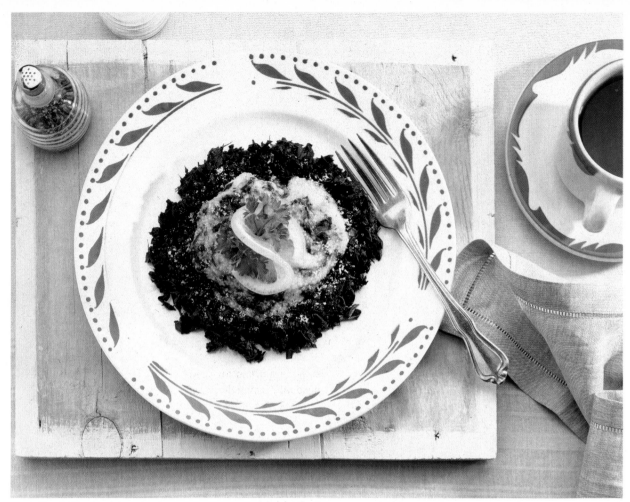

Semolina with Greens and Garlic

SEMOLINA WITH GREENS AND GARLIC

Dark leafy greens are not only good sources of vitamin A, iron and potassium, but are among the best non-dairy sources of calcium as well.

1 tablespoon olive oil	125 g (4 oz) semolina
8 garlic cloves, crushed	¼ teaspoon salt
500 g (1 lb) finely shredded	¼ teaspoon black pepper
beetroot greens or kale	1 egg, beaten
4 tablespoons chopped parsley,	45 g (1½ oz) freshly grated
plus 4 sprigs	Parmesan
60 cl (1 pint) skimmed milk	Lemon slices, for garnish

CALORIES per serving	300
50% Carbohydrate	40 g
23% Protein	17 g
27% Fat	9 g
CALCIUM	504 mg
IRON	5 mg
SODIUM	353 mg

Heat the oil in a medium-sized saucepan, add the garlic and sauté for 2 minutes, or until fragrant. Add the greens, parsley and 3 tablespoons of water, cover and cook gently for 10 to 12 minutes or until the greens are cooked, stirring occasionally. Bring the milk to the boil in a pan set over medium-high heat. Stir in the semolina with a wooden spoon and cook for 3 to 4 minutes, stirring all the time until the mixture thickens. Beat in the salt, pepper, egg and 30 g (1 oz) of the Parmesan. Spoon the semolina mixture into the centre of four plates, and surround with the greens. Sprinkle with the remaining Parmesan; garnish with lemon twists and parsley.

Makes 4 servings

PINEAPPLE-OAT MUFFINS ▼

Wrap the muffins individually and freeze them, then thaw one at a time as a portable breakfast. If you usually stop en route to work for a croissant or pastry, you will save minutes as well as calories.

300 g (10 oz) plain flour
2 teaspoons baking powder
2¼ teaspoons ground ginger
2¼ teaspoons ground cinnamon
3 large eggs, lightly beaten
6 slices unsweetened dried
    pineapple, finely chopped

17.5 cl (6 fl oz) pineapple juice
4 tablespoons honey
4 teaspoons vegetable oil
1½ teaspoons pure vanilla
    extract
75 g (2½ oz) rolled oats

CALORIES per muffin	185
72% Carbohydrate	34 g
11% Protein	5 g
17% Fat	4 g
CALCIUM	60 mg
IRON	2 mg
SODIUM	90 mg

Preheat the oven to 200°C (400°F or Mark 6). Lightly oil 12 deep bun tins or line them with paper liners; set aside. Sift the flour, baking powder, ginger and cinnamon into a medium-sized bowl; set aside. In a large bowl, stir together the eggs, pineapple, pineapple juice, honey, oil and vanilla. Stir in the sifted dry ingredients and the oats and stir just until combined: do not overmix. Divide the batter among the tins and bake for 20 minutes, or until a toothpick inserted in the centre of a muffin comes out clean. Transfer the muffins to a rack to cool. If you are freezing the muffins, wrap them individually in plastic film when completely cooled. Makes 12 muffins

JOHNNY CAKES WITH BLUEBERRY SAUCE

Johnny cakes are light, crisp cornmeal griddle cakes made without eggs or butter. The cooked berries in this recipe are naturally sweet without added sugar, making them a healthier topping than syrups that are virtually pure sugar.

225 g (7½ oz) fresh blueberries,
    washed, or frozen unsweetened
    blueberries, thawed
2 tablespoons orange juice
½ teaspoon grated orange rind

125 g (4 oz) cornmeal
Pinch of salt
4 tablespoons skimmed milk
1 tablespoon vegetable oil

A rtificial sweeteners may not help you lose weight; in fact, they may hinder your efforts at weight control. The sweeteners do not satisfy hunger, and in some people they actually stimulate feelings of hunger. A study has shown that long-time users of artificial sweeteners are more likely to gain weight in the course of a year than people who do not use the sweeteners and, in addition, they are more likely to gain more weight (more than 16 per cent of body weight) than non-users.

For the sauce, combine the blueberries, orange juice and orange rind in a medium-sized non-reactive saucepan and cook over medium heat, stirring and mashing the berries with a wooden spoon, for 7 to 10 minutes, or until the sauce is thick and syrupy. Remove the pan from the heat and cover it to keep the sauce warm; set aside.

Bring a small saucepan of water to the boil. In a large bowl, stir together the cornmeal and salt. Add 30 cl (½ pint) of boiling water and mix well, then stir in the milk. Heat the oil in a heavy non-stick frying pan over medium heat. Using a scant 4 tablespoons of batter for each, make four griddle cakes. Cook the cakes for 3 minutes, or until they are golden on the bottom, then turn them and cook for another 3 to 5 minutes, or until golden and crisp. Transfer the cakes to a plate. Use the remaining batter to make another four griddle cakes in the same fashion and place them on a second plate. Pour the blueberry sauce over the johnny cakes and serve. Makes 2 servings

CALORIES per serving	390
74% Carbohydrate	73 g
7% Protein	7 g
19% Fat	8 g
CALCIUM	51 mg
IRON	2 mg
SODIUM	89 mg

GINGERBREAD-BROWN RICE GRIDDLE CAKES ▼

When you include low-fat dairy products such as buttermilk and low-fat ricotta cheese in your breakfast dishes, you keep your calorie, fat and cholesterol intakes low and get plenty of calcium as well.

90 g (3 oz) brown rice	¾ teaspoon ground cinnamon
2 tablespoons lemon juice	½ teaspoon ground cloves
2 tablespoons honey	17.5 cl (6 fl oz) buttermilk
2 teaspoons cornflour	3 tablespoons molasses
150 g (5 oz) plain flour	2 egg whites
30 g (1 oz) chopped walnuts	1 tablespoon grated fresh ginger
1 teaspoon baking powder	root
½ teaspoon bicarbonate of soda	60 g (2 oz) low-fat ricotta cheese

Bring 30 cl (½ pint) of water to the boil in a small saucepan over medium heat. Add the rice, cover the pan, reduce the heat to low and cook for 30 minutes, or until the rice is just tender and the water is absorbed. Remove the pan from the heat and allow it to cool until the rice is just warm.

Meanwhile, for the sauce, stir together the lemon juice, honey, cornflour and 2 tablespoons of water in a small saucepan. Bring the sauce to the boil over medium heat, stirring constantly, and boil for 30 seconds, or until the sauce thickens. Remove the pan from the heat and set aside to cool.

Stir together the flour, walnuts, baking powder, bicarbonate of soda, cinnamon and cloves in a large bowl and make a well in the centre. Pour in the buttermilk, molasses, egg whites and ginger and stir until combined. Stir the rice to break it up, then add it to the batter and stir just until combined.

Preheat the oven to 95°C (200°F or Mark ¼). Heat a medium-sized non-stick frying pan over medium-low heat. Using 2 tablespoons of batter for each, make three griddle cakes. Cook for 3 minutes, or until bubbles form on the tops of the cakes, then turn and cook for 3 minutes, or until golden. Transfer the cakes to an ovenproof platter, cover with foil and place in the oven to keep warm. Make another five batches of griddle cakes in the same way.

Fold the ricotta into the sauce; divide the griddle cakes among six plates and top each serving with a heaped tablespoon of sauce.   Makes 6 servings

CALORIES per serving	245
71% Carbohydrate	44 g
12% Protein	7 g
17% Fat	5 g
CALCIUM	189 mg
IRON	3 mg
SODIUM	215 mg

CARROT-BUTTERMILK SHAKE

This drink combines carrots and apricots, both rich in vitamin A, with low-fat buttermilk, which adds high-quality protein. The apple, carrots and nuts provide fibre and give this filling meal in a glass a rich, thick texture.

1 crisp red-skinned apple	½ teaspoon grated fresh ginger
(about 150 g/5 oz)	root
150 g (5 oz) cooked sliced carrots	35 cl (12 fl oz) buttermilk
2 tablespoons chopped walnuts	25 cl (8 fl oz) apricot nectar
2 tablespoons dark brown sugar	2 ice cubes

Peel and core the apple and cut it into large chunks. Place the apple and all the remaining ingredients in a food processor or blender and process until smooth. Pour the shake into two tall glasses and serve.   Makes 2 servings

CALORIES per serving	315
71% Carbohydrate	59 g
11% Protein	9 g
18% Fat	7 g
CALCIUM	267 mg
IRON	2 mg
SODIUM	253 mg

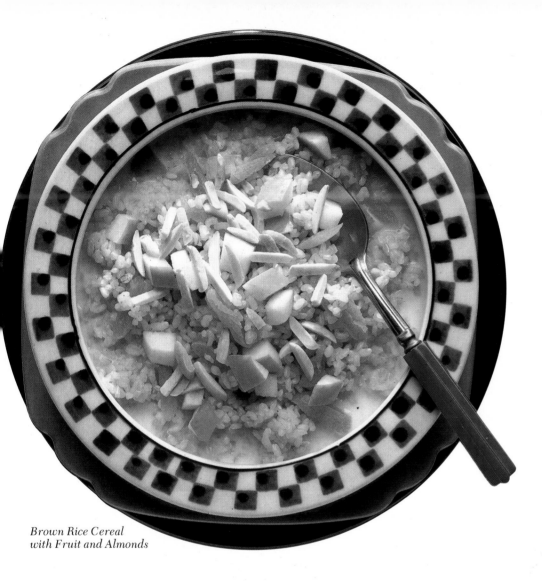

*Brown Rice Cereal
with Fruit and Almonds*

BROWN RICE CEREAL WITH FRUIT AND ALMONDS

Brown rice, apricots, almonds and an unpeeled apple provide a fibre-rich breakfast with none of the refined sweeteners (sugar, dextrose or corn syrup) usually added to packaged breakfast cereals.

375 g (13 oz) brown rice
¼ teaspoon ground allspice
Pinch of salt
60 g (2 oz) dried apricots, cut into thin strips

1 Golden Delicious apple
60 g (2 oz) slivered toasted almonds
50 cl (16 fl oz) semi-skimmed milk

CALORIES per serving	345
67% Carbohydrate	62 g
11% Protein	9 g
22% Fat	8 g
CALCIUM	145 mg
IRON	2 mg
SODIUM	51 mg

Place the rice, allspice, salt and 1 litre (1¾ pints) of water in a medium-sized saucepan and bring to the boil over medium heat. Cover the pan, reduce the heat to low and cook for 40 minutes, or until the rice is tender and the water is absorbed. Add the apricots and cook for another 5 minutes. Core and chop the apple. Divide the cereal among six bowls, sprinkle with the almonds and apple, and pour some milk over each serving.   Makes 6 servings

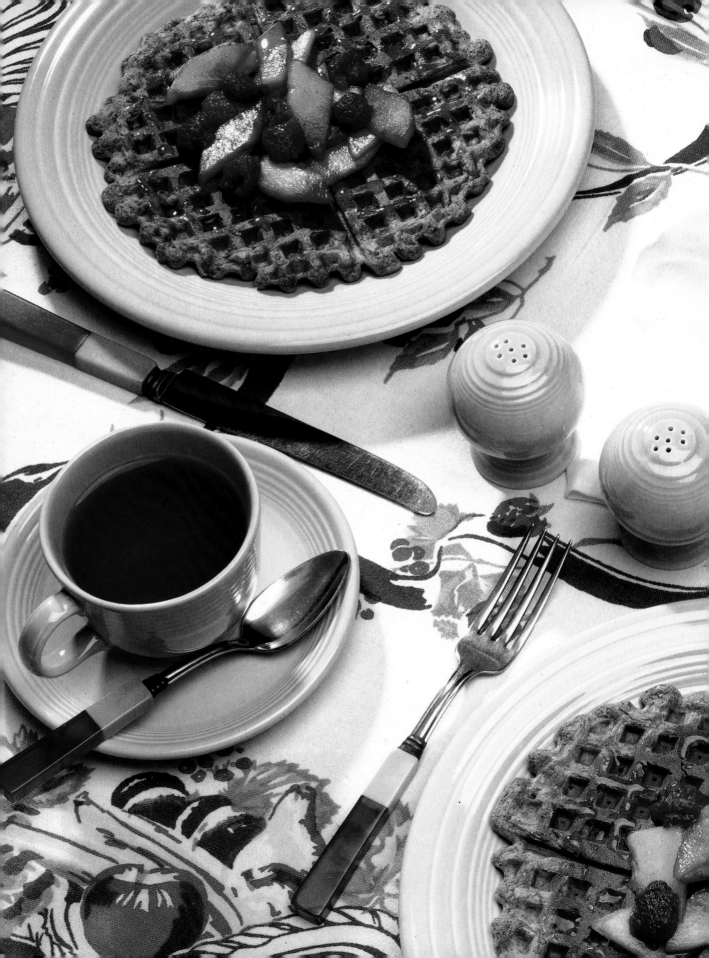

BUCKWHEAT-WILD RICE WAFFLES

Egg whites can be substituted for whole eggs in many waffle and griddle cake recipes, thereby cutting fat and cholesterol. These waffles have a hearty flavour thanks to the combination of buckwheat and wild rice.

CALORIES per serving	300
70% Carbohydrate	53 g
11% Protein	9 g
19% Fat	7 g
CALCIUM	174 mg
IRON	2 mg
SODIUM	293 mg

150 g (5 oz) plain flour
75 g (2½ oz) light buckwheat
   flour
2 teaspoons baking powder
¼ teaspoon salt
3 tablespoons honey
2 tablespoons vegetable oil
35 cl (12 fl oz) semi-skimmed milk
3 egg whites

3 tablespoons wild rice, cooked
   and cooled
150 g (5 oz) cantaloupe melon
   flesh, thinly sliced
125 g (4 oz) fresh raspberries or
   frozen unsweetened raspberries,
   thawed
3 tablespoons pure maple syrup

In a large bowl, stir together the flours, baking powder and salt and make a well in the centre. Pour in the honey and oil and mix until blended. Add the milk and stir until the batter is fairly smooth; set aside.

Preheat the oven to 95°C (200°F or Mark ¼). Lightly oil a non-stick waffle iron and preheat it. In a large bowl, beat the egg whites using an electric mixer until soft peaks form. Gently fold the egg whites into the batter, then fold in the wild rice. Pour 25 cl (8 fl oz) of batter into the waffle iron and cook for 2 to 3 minutes, or according to the manufacturer's instructions, until the waffle is golden. Transfer the waffle to an ovenproof platter and place it in the oven to keep warm. Using the remaining batter, make five more waffles in the same fashion. (Do not re-oil the hot waffle iron.)

Divide the waffles among six plates, top with the melon and raspberries, and dribble the maple syrup over each waffle.   Makes 6 servings

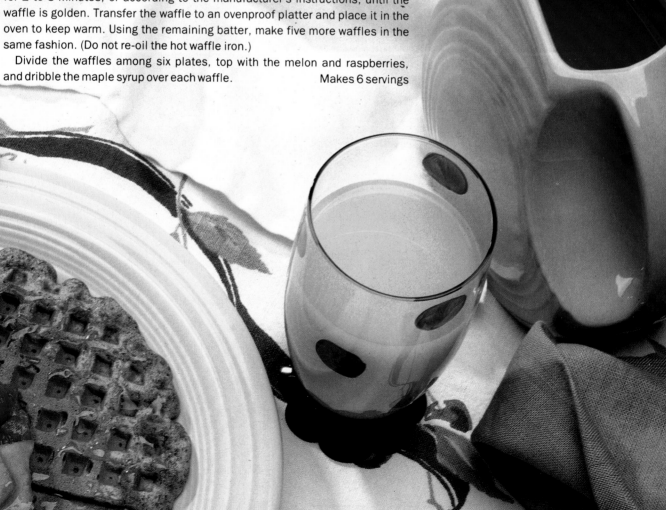

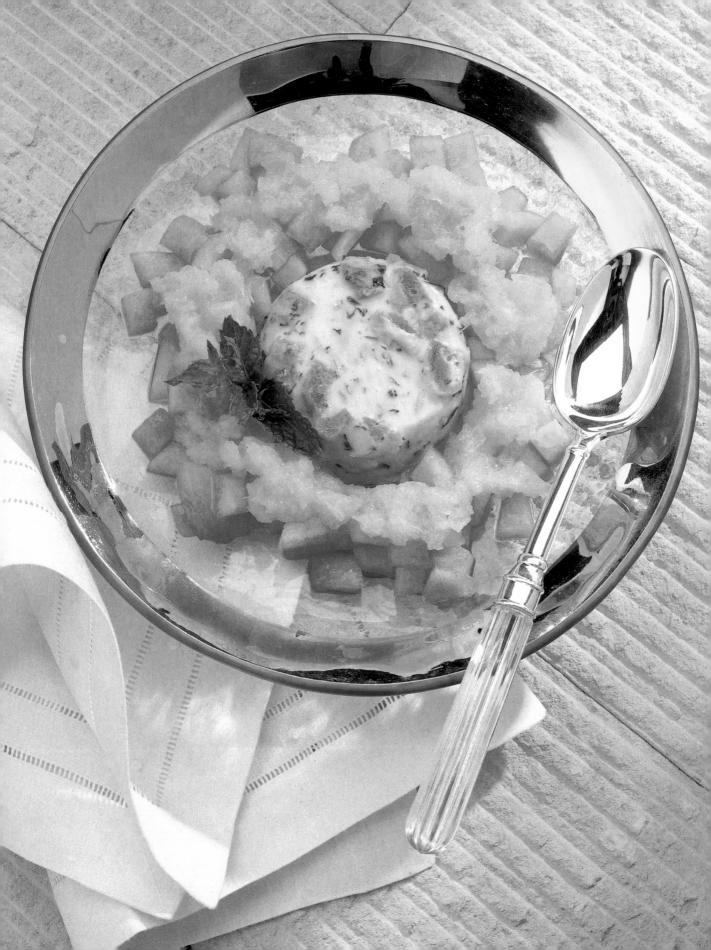

RICOTTA MOUSSE WITH CHUNKY PINEAPPLE SAUCE

This mousse, with its combination of fruit and low-fat dairy products, is a pleasant breakfast and provides a day's supply of vitamins A and C.

1 egg yolk
12.5 cl (4 fl oz) semi-skimmed
  milk
4 tablespoons sugar
7 g (¼ oz) powdered gelatine
1 teaspoon grated orange rind
250 g (8 oz) low-fat ricotta cheese
12.5 cl (4 fl oz) orange juice
¼ teaspoon pure vanilla extract

30 g (1 oz) chopped fresh mint
  leaves, plus sprigs for garnish
30 g (1 oz) dried apricots, chopped
350 g (12 oz) drained juice-packed
  pineapple chunks
6 tablespoons lemon juice
1 teaspoon grated lemon rind
1 cantaloupe melon, peeled, seeded
  and chopped (about 600 g/1¼ lb)

CALORIES per serving	325
65% Carbohydrate	55 g
15% Protein	13 g
20% Fat	8 g
CALCIUM	257 mg
IRON	2 mg
SODIUM	117 mg

Bring water to a simmer in the bottom of a double boiler; the simmering water should not touch the top pan. Place the egg yolk and milk in the top pan and cook, whisking constantly, for 10 minutes, or until the mixture begins to thicken slightly. Add the sugar, gelatine and orange rind, and cook, stirring constantly, for 8 minutes, or until the mixture is quite thick. Transfer to a medium-sized bowl and set aside to cool for about 15 minutes.

Meanwhile, place the ricotta, orange juice and vanilla in a food processor or blender and process for 1 minute. Add the chopped mint and process for another 20 seconds. Fold the ricotta mixture into the gelatine mixture, then fold in the apricots until well combined. Spoon the mousse into four 12.5 cl (4 fl oz) moulds, cover and refrigerate for at least 1 hour, or overnight.

For the sauce, combine the pineapple, lemon juice and lemon rind in a small saucepan and cook over medium heat for 5 minutes, then transfer the mixture to a food processor or blender and process for 10 seconds, or just until roughly chopped. Cover and refrigerate the sauce until ready to serve.

To turn out the mousses, dip each mould in a bowl of hot water for 10 to 15 seconds, then invert it on a plate. Surround each mousse with one quarter of the melon and spoon some of the pineapple sauce over the melon. Garnish with the mint sprigs. Makes 4 servings

R *ather than concentrating on those foods you must avoid, look for less familiar but nutritious foods to add variety to your diet. Many of the more exotic fruits — such as papayas, mangoes, kiwi fruits, pomegranates, Asia pears, star fruits, kumquats and passion fruits — are good low-calorie sources of vitamins A and C and potassium as well as fibre. These fruits are becoming more widely available in supermarkets.*

FRUIT GAZPACHO COOLER

Some commercial soft drinks contain fruit juice and modest amounts of vitamin C: this sharp refresher has nearly the full daily requirement of vitamin C and a good amount of vitamin A — and has no refined sugar or artificial sweetener.

45 g (1½ oz) washed, stemmed
  seedless grapes
12.5 cl (4 fl oz) low-sodium tomato
  juice

4 tablespoons freshly squeezed
  orange juice
1 tablespoon soured cream

CALORIES per serving	110
66% Carbohydrate	19 g
7% Protein	2 g
27% Fat	3 g
CALCIUM	39 mg
IRON	1 mg
SODIUM	21 mg

Spread the grapes on a small plate and freeze them for 2 hours, or until frozen solid. Place the tomato juice and orange juice in a blender and start the machine, then add the grapes and process until coarsely chopped. Pour the drink into a glass, top with the soured cream and serve. Makes 1 serving

◁ *Ricotta Mousse with Chunky Pineapple Sauce*

Mid-Morning Snacks

OATMEAL BANANA BARS

CALORIES per bar	75
75% Carbohydrate	15 g
10% Protein	2 g
15% Fat	1 g
CALCIUM	11 mg
IRON	1 mg
SODIUM	7 mg

This healthy snack cake is sweetened with banana, currants, unsweetened apple juice — and just one tablespoon of sugar.

1 tablespoon soft margarine
1 tablespoon brown sugar
75 g (2½ oz) rolled oats
¼ teaspoon ground cinnamon
60 g (2 oz) wholemeal flour

12.5 cl (4 fl oz) apple juice
½ teaspoon pure vanilla extract
1 banana, mashed
45 g (1½ oz) dried currants

Preheat the oven to 180°C (350°F or Mark 4). Lightly oil a 20 cm (8 inch) square baking tin. In a medium-sized bowl, beat together the margarine and sugar until creamy. Stir in the oats and cinnamon until combined, then add the flour and stir to combine. Mix the apple juice, vanilla and 12.5 cl (4 fl oz) of warm water in a small bowl, then add this mixture to the dry ingredients and stir well. Stir in the banana and currants. Spread the dough in the prepared tin, smoothing the top with a rubber spatula, and bake for about 1 hour, or until the top is golden. Let the cake cool in the tin on a rack. Cut the cake into quarters, then cut each quarter into three bars.   Makes 12 bars

Rye-Cheese Biscuits

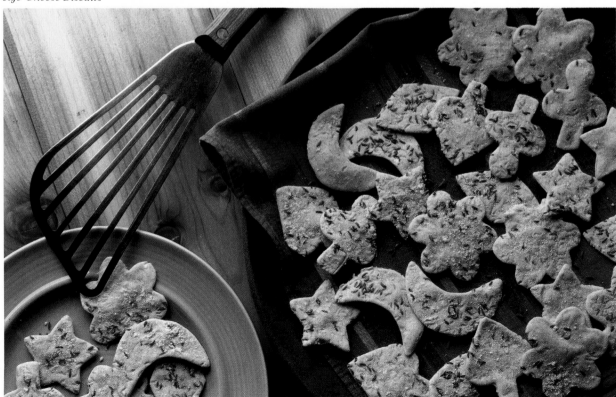

CRANBERRY POACHED PEARS WITH YOGURT

Low-calorie diets are often deficient in iron. Cranberry juice contains iron, and this dish also supplies vitamin C, which helps the body use the iron.

CALORIES per serving	165
73% Carbohydrate	32 g
10% Protein	4 g
17% Fat	3 g
CALCIUM	146 mg
IRON	4 mg
SODIUM	46 mg

25 cl (8 fl oz) unsweetened
   cranberry juice
1 teaspoon sugar
1 teaspoon grated lemon rind
½ teaspoon grated orange rind
½ teaspoon pure vanilla extract
1 cinnamon stick

2 whole cloves
1 large pear, peeled, halved and
   cored
12.5 cl (4 fl oz) plain low-fat
   yogurt
1 tablespoon toasted sesame
   seeds

In a medium-sized non-reactive saucepan, combine the cranberry juice, sugar, lemon rind, orange rind, vanilla, cinnamon stick and cloves, and bring to the boil over medium-high heat. Reduce the heat to low and simmer the mixture for 5 minutes. Add the pear halves and simmer for 15 minutes, turning occasionally. Remove the pan from the heat; remove and discard the cinnamon and cloves. Transfer the pear halves and poaching liquid to a small bowl and set aside to cool to room temperature, basting the pears often with the liquid if they are not completely immersed. Refrigerate for at least 30 minutes, or until well chilled. To serve, spoon 4 tablespoons of yogurt over each pear half and sprinkle with the sesame seeds.   Makes 2 servings

RYE-CHEESE BISCUITS

Instead of buying a packet of fatty, highly salted snacks, keep these low-calorie biscuits on hand to assuage the craving for something crunchy.

CALORIES per serving	85
70% Carbohydrate	15 g
9% Protein	2 g
21% Fat	2 g
CALCIUM	21 mg
IRON	1 mg
SODIUM	129 mg

150 g (5 oz) plain flour,
   approximately
50 g (1¾ oz) light rye flour
½ teaspoon salt

15 g (½ oz) unsalted butter or
   margarine, well chilled
1½ teaspoons caraway seeds
2 tablespoons grated Parmesan

In a medium-sized bowl, stir together the plain flour, rye flour and salt. Cut the butter into pieces, then with your fingers rub it into the dry ingredients until the mixture resembles coarse crumbs. Add the caraway seeds and 12.5 cl (4 fl oz) of cold water and stir until the dough begins to gather into a mass, then form it into a ball with your hands. Flatten the dough into a disc, wrap it in plastic film and allow it to rest at room temperature for 30 minutes.

  Preheat the oven to 150°C (300°F or Mark 2). Lightly flour the work surface and a rolling pin. Roll out the dough to a thickness of 1.5 mm (1/16 inch). Using 5 cm (2 inch) biscuit cutters in various shapes, cut out about 60 biscuits, cutting them as close together as possible. (Do not reroll any excess dough; it will be tough when baked.) Place the biscuits on a lightly oiled baking sheet, sprinkle with the grated Parmesan and bake for 12 minutes, or until crisp and lightly browned. Transfer the biscuits to racks to cool, then store in an airtight container for up to a week.   Makes 10 servings

Note: instead of cutting the dough with biscuit cutters, you can use a ruler and a sharp knife to cut it into 6 cm (2½ inch) squares.

RICE CAKES WITH VEGETABLE-CHEESE SPREAD

CALORIES per serving	85
63% Carbohydrate	13 g
19% Protein	4 g
18% Fat	2 g
CALCIUM	75 mg
IRON	1 mg
SODIUM	45 mg

A herbed ricotta and vegetable topping is a fine nutritional complement to crisp rice cakes, which are made from whole grains with no added fat.

125 g (4 oz) low-fat ricotta cheese
250 g (8 oz) carrots, grated
125 g (4 oz) sweet red pepper, finely chopped
30 g (1 oz) celery, finely chopped
3 tablespoons chopped spring onions

2 tablespoons chopped parsley
½ teaspoon chopped fresh thyme, or ¼ teaspoon dried thyme
1 tablespoon lemon juice
¼ teaspoon grated lemon rind
6 rice cakes

Purée the ricotta in a food processor or blender until completely smooth. Stir in the vegetables, herbs, lemon juice and rind, and stir until well combined. Spread the mixture on the rice cakes and serve.   Makes 6 servings

RYE AND CRACKED WHEAT FLATBREAD

CALORIES per serving	100
72% Carbohydrate	18 g
11% Protein	3 g
17% Fat	2 g
CALCIUM	12 mg
IRON	1 mg
SODIUM	77 mg

Packaged savoury biscuits may derive up to 60 per cent of their calories from highly saturated fats such as lard, palm kernel oil and coconut oil. However, most of the cooking oils sold for home use are low in saturated fat. Sunflower and safflower oils are among the lowest.

3 tablespoons cracked wheat
¾ teaspoon dried yeast
1½ tablespoons brown sugar
75 g (2½ oz) plain flour, approximately

75 g (2½ oz) rye flour
2 teaspoons dried skimmed milk
1 tablespoon vegetable oil
1 egg white
¼ teaspoon salt

L ittle changes can add up: if you drink three cups of coffee a day and have a teaspoon of cream in each, giving up the cream — with no other changes in your diet — would cause you to lose nearly 2 kilograms in a year. Or, if you gave up a tablespoon of butter every day for a year, you would lose more than 4 kilograms.

Place the cracked wheat in a small bowl, add 4 tablespoons of boiling water and set aside to soak for 5 minutes. Combine the yeast, sugar and 4 tablespoons of warm water (40-45°C/105-115°F) in a small bowl and set aside for 5 minutes.

Combine the flours, dried milk, 2 teaspoons of the oil, the egg white, cracked wheat and ⅛ teaspoon of the salt in a food processor. Start the machine, then pour the yeast mixture through the feed tube. Process for 40 seconds; the dough should form a ball. Transfer to a bowl, cover with a tea towel and set aside in a warm place to rise for 50 minutes, or until doubled in bulk.

Preheat the oven to 200°C (400°F or Mark 6). Lightly flour the work surface. Knock back the dough and roll it out to a 25 by 40 cm (10 by 16 inch) rectangle. Cut the dough in half to form two 12.5 by 40 cm (5 by 16 inch) rectangles. Transfer one to a baking sheet and prick it all over with a fork; cut the dough widthwise into six equal strips, then cut each strip diagonally to form 12 triangles. Separate the triangles slightly. Repeat with the second sheet of dough. Bake in the centre of the oven for 8 to 10 minutes, or until golden. Brush the hot flatbreads with the remaining oil, then sprinkle with the remaining salt. Cool on a rack, or serve them warm.   Makes 8 servings

Note: the cooled flatbreads should be stored in an airtight container; they will keep for up to a week. Reheat them briefly in a warm oven before serving.

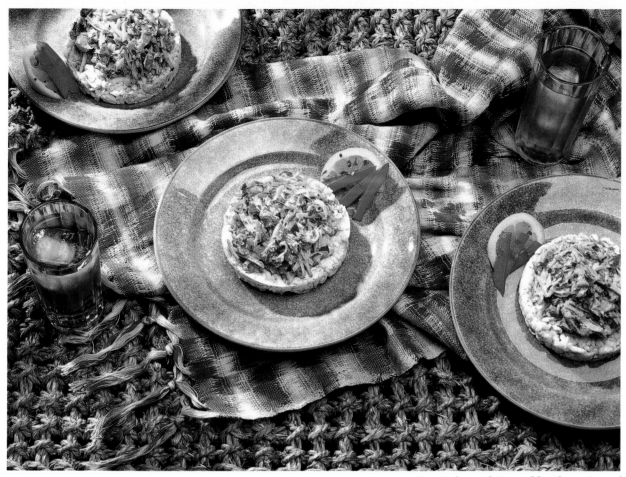

Rice Cakes with Vegetable-Cheese Spread

WHOLEMEAL CRANBERRY MUFFINS

Cranberries are low in calories — 150 g (5 oz) contain just 25 — but contribute to the fibre content of these wholemeal muffins, making them a healthy, filling snack.

CALORIES per muffin	140
65% Carbohydrate	23 g
9% Protein	3 g
26% Fat	4 g
CALCIUM	69 mg
IRON	1 mg
SODIUM	141 mg

125 g (4 oz) wholemeal flour
75 g (2½ oz) plain flour
2 teaspoons baking powder
½ teaspoon ground cinnamon
Pinch of salt
12.5 cl (4 fl oz) skimmed milk

60 g (2 oz) soft margarine, melted
  and cooled
4 tablespoons honey
1 large egg, lightly beaten
150 g (5 oz) cranberries, coarsely
  chopped

Preheat the oven to 200°C (400°F or Mark 6). Lightly oil 10 deep bun tins or line them with paper liners; set aside. In a large bowl, stir together the flours, baking powder, cinnamon and salt. In a small bowl, stir together the milk, margarine, honey and egg. Add the milk mixture to the dry ingredients and stir vigorously for 30 seconds. Stir in the cranberries. Divide the batter among the tins and bake for 30 minutes, or until the tops are golden and a toothpick inserted in a muffin comes out clean.   Makes 10 muffins

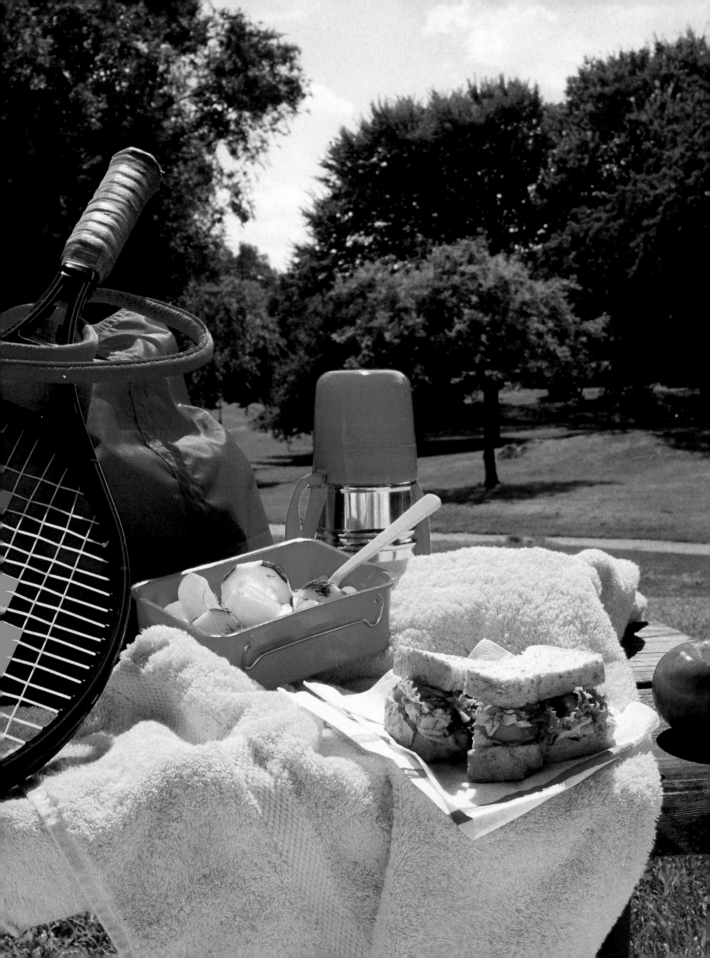

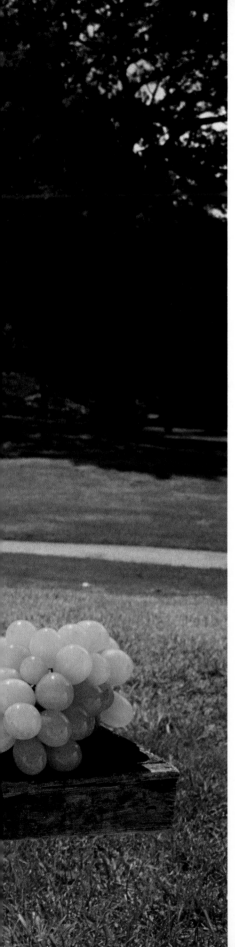

Lunch

Avoiding the unwanted calories in sandwiches and at salad bars

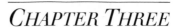

For the midday meal, many weight-conscious people face the problem of choosing foods from a cafeteria, snack bar or fast-food restaurant where they have little or no control over the ingredients in a dish or its preparation. Consider sandwiches: those made in a snack bar are typically packed with cold meats that derive up to 80 per cent of their calories from fat. Salami, for example, has almost 500 calories per 100 grams and a generous salami sandwich may contain that weight of meat. Such a sandwich might be served with a side order of coleslaw or potato salad, both of which generally contain large amounts of high-fat mayonnaise. In fact, dressings and side dishes accompanying a sandwich can be the source of hidden calories at lunch. A 90 gram hamburger in a bun has a fairly modest 300 to 350 calories. But if the hamburger is topped with a mayonnaise-based sauce, condiments or cheese, or if it is served with French fries or deep-fried onion rings, the calories you consume for your lunch may be more than double those of a plain hamburger.

75

▼ Most of the main-dish recipes in this chapter have from 300 to 395 calories per serving. Certain recipes, marked with a triangle, are extra-low in calories — between 140 and 275 per serving. These can be eaten as main dishes or they can be combined with other foods. The desserts in this chapter contain fewer than 275 calories. The mid-afternoon snacks in the section following the main dishes all have fewer than 200 calories.

In their quest for a lighter, more nutritious lunch, growing numbers of people are turning to salad bars. Despite their healthy image, however, many salad bars offer foods full of unexpected calories. Alongside low-calorie vegetables and fruits, you are likely to find bacon bits, diced ham, olives, avocados and cheese — all of which would add a large number of calories to a low-fat meal. The oil-based dressings you can add to salad-bar ingredients can raise the calorie count by 50 to 100 calories per spoonful. A university study comparing students who ate a salad-bar lunch with those who ate a cafeteria hot meal found that the salad-bar patrons consumed more calories than the others and that a greater percentage of their calories came from fat.

The best weight-control strategy for lunch is to make your own meal, which will also ensure its nutritional value. You can draw on a variety of foods — fruits, vegetables, low-fat cheeses and yogurt, fish, pasta, grains, pulses and poultry — that will fill you up without adding excess calories. Instead of having an overstuffed processed meat sandwich, for example, use skinless turkey breast or chicken, both of which have about half the calories of luncheon meat or salami. Tuna packed in water, not in oil, is also a good choice. You can reduce the fat content of a sandwich even further by supplementing a small amount of meat with vegetables, as in the vegetable-and-chicken pitta sandwich on page 98. And instead of adding butter, margarine or mayonnaise, substitute low-fat yogurt, mustard or horseradish.

Salads make excellent low-calorie, nutrient-rich lunches. Instead of the standard mixed green salad, you can use denser, more filling ingredients, as in the Florida Halibut Salad on page 92, which combines fish with asparagus, oranges and a sweet potato, or the Green Salad with Chicken and Mangoes on page 87. The oil that is contained in conventional dressings can immediately turn any salad into a high-calorie dish, so dress your salad with vinegar and herbs, lemon juice or low-fat yogurt, and try to keep the amount of oil to a teaspoon or less per serving. A good example is the dressing for the Apple, Fennel and Pasta salad given on page 99, which uses balsamic vinegar and oil in proportions that are almost the reverse of many oil-heavy dressings served in restaurants and at salad bars.

One of the best lunchtime choices for the weight-conscious is soup, which has a lower caloric density than most solid foods and which tends to take longer to eat. Research indicates that people who eat soup tend to feel full before they have consumed many calories. In one study, subjects who were served low-calorie tomato soup reported feeling full on the same amount of soup as subjects who ate a higher-calorie soup. Yet the first group consumed approximately one tenth of the calories consumed by the second group. The Curried Vegetable Soup on page 91 and Oriental Scallop Soup on page 88 use low-fat ingredients that are substantial enough to keep you from overeating, and they are also low in sodium, which is often added to commercial canned soups in the form of salt and monosodium glutamate (MSG).

Choosing a Beverage

Even if you are conscientious about what you eat at lunchtime, your attempt to control your weight may be foiled if you do not pay equal attention to what you drink. The following guidelines point out the calorie content of various beverages and their effect on your diet.

◆ Water is one of the best thirst-quenchers, whether you drink it in the form of club soda, sparkling mineral water, mineral water or plain tap water. It relieves your thirst as effectively as other types of beverages, or even better, and it has no calories. Club sodas and many mineral waters generally contain sodium, but salt-free varieties are available.

◆ Soft drinks are among the worst drinks for those seeking to control their weight. Non-diet soft drinks typically contain 140 to 150 calories per 35 centilitre can, and 99 per cent of these calories may come from sugar. Diet soft drinks that contain the artificial sweetener aspartame have no calories, but they may have serious side effects for sensitive people.

◆ Fruit juices are often good sources of vitamins and minerals, but they contain a significant number of calories. A 25 centilitre glass of orange juice, for example, has about 110 calories, and a glass of canned pineapple juice has 140. You can retain much of the taste of fruit juice while reducing its calories by diluting it with sparkling mineral water.

◆ Alcoholic beverages tend to be high in calories and low in nutrients. There are about 150 calories in a 35 centilitre bottle of beer. Light beers contain about 100 calories, and a 17.5 centilitre glass of wine contains about 160. Hard liquors are even more concentrated: one tot (4.5 centilitres) of 70% proof gin, vodka or whisky contains 95 calories, and with a mixer, you may consume more than 200 calories. There is also some indication that the alcohol contained in one or two drinks can increase your appetite. Therefore, if you do drink alcoholic beverages, restrict your intake and drink during a meal rather than beforehand.

◆ Coffee and tea usually have fewer than five calories per cup. But when you add whole milk, cream or a non-dairy creamer — which is high in saturated fat — you are adding some 25 calories per serving. And pre-sweetened teas or coffees contain many more calories. The caffeine in coffee and tea can also cause such side effects as irritability, headaches and nervousness when consumed in excess, so it is a good idea to drink no more than two cups a day.

Skipping lunch is one weight-control strategy you should not adopt. Because of work-related pressures and because lunch breaks can be short, you may be tempted not to eat. But not eating in the middle of the day may encourage bingeing or overeating in the afternoon and evening. Lunch skippers are likely to resort to eating a succession of snacks such as potato crisps, biscuits, chocolates, sweets and other foods that are typically high in sugar and sodium, refined flours and saturated fats. Having lunch not only helps you avoid overeating later, but boosts your energy level during the afternoon. If you feel like a snack mid-afternoon, choose one from those recommended on pages 78-79. You can also make one of the recipes on pages 102-107 as a satisfying alternative to more conventional snacks.

Controlling Cravings

The impulses to eat food that you want but do not need can be troublesome when you are following a reduced-calorie diet. Even scientists who have studied the subject cannot explain why people have sudden and sometimes uncontrollable urges for certain foods or taste sensations. Researchers have established, however, that many cravings have psychological, rather than physical, causes.

Your appetite for food is a combination of your body chemistry, the functioning of your senses and the psychological connotations that a particular food may have for you. The secretion of the female hormone progesterone, for example, may account for the cravings that women experience during menstruation and pregnancy. One study found that women consume 30 per cent more carbohydrates during menstruation than they do at any other time during the rest of their menstrual cycle.

Opinion is divided on a possible link between carbohydrate cravings and a substance in the brain called serotonin. Some scientists suspect that eating carbohydrates can help certain people to overcome anxiety or depression. Ongoing research may clarify whether a person's carbohydrate consumption does prompt the brain to make enough serotonin to elevate his or her mood.

Why certain tastes have special appeal to people is not well understood. A craving for sugar may be genetic; the same may be true of salt, which, after sugar, is the most commonly used food additive. But some researchers think that cravings are more a matter of eating habits than of taste appeal.

Examining your own emotional attachments to food may be the best approach to controlling cravings that are stress-related. For example, if you tend to eat a chocolate bar, or biscuit or another form of sweet when a stressful situation confronts you, it may be that a parent always gave you sweets to calm you down when you were upset as a child. Once you have recognized the origin of a bad habit, you may be able to break it relatively easily.

One of the best ways to handle cravings is to monitor and control your snacks, since most weight-loss plans aim to minimize between-meal eating. The chart opposite shows a wide range of recommended snacks. If you consume an afternoon snack at your office, choose items listed in the "excellent" and "acceptable" categories, rather than those from a bakery or sweet counter.

A number of other diet-orientated strategies follow:

● Identify the specific food that you crave. Do not simply eat whatever is available until you feel full.

● Try to satisfy a craving for sweets with a piece of fruit, a glass of fruit juice or a low-sugar biscuit. An average sized apple has 80 to 90 calories; a typical chewy chocolate bar has at least 250 calories.

● To satisfy a craving for salt, drink a glass of low-sodium tomato or other vegetable juice. Lightly salted, air-popped popcorn is a good alternative to heavily salted nuts and crisps if you feel like a snack.

● Eat foods high in fibre and complex carbohydrates before you indulge in a less wholesome food you crave. A slice or two of wholemeal bread or a plate of raw vegetables will help fill you up and may distract you from sugary or salty snacks.

HOW SNACKS STACK UP

Eating between meals can be an effective hunger-controlling element in a weight-control plan. But fatty snacks violate the basic tenets of a low-calorie diet. The examples below, grouped according to fat content, show what snacks are best.

EXCELLENT

low-fat cottage cheese
fresh fruit
low-fat plain yogurt with fruit
rye crispbread
plain breadsticks
raw vegetables
rice cake
unbuttered popcorn, air-popped
unsweetened cereal with skimmed milk
wholemeal bread with all-fruit preserves

ACCEPTABLE

rye crispbread with low-fat mozzarella
corn bread
dried fruit
dry roasted nuts, no salt
flavoured jelly with fresh fruit
flavoured ices
gingersnaps
low-fat vanilla yogurt
pretzels
ricotta cheese and rye crackers
white bread toast with jam

NOT RECOMMENDED

brownie
chocolate bar
chocolate chip cookies
chocolate pudding
cream-filled doughnut
croissant with butter
Danish pastry
éclair
ice cream
milk shake
potato crisps

Body Toning

As you are losing weight, exercises to shape and tone your muscles will help you to develop an aesthetically pleasing physique. Firm, strong muscles also contribute to your actual weight loss; as your muscle mass increases with strength training, your calorie expenditure is accelerated. Even at rest, muscle tissue burns more calories than fat tissue.

As a result of inactivity, however, many people lose muscle mass as they gain fat round their waist and thighs. Weakened musculature also affects posture. When your stomach muscles sag, they may contribute to excessive curvature of the back or spine, forcing the back to hold up more than its share of body weight, resulting in lower back pain.

The exercises on these two pages can restore your body's pleasing proportions, make your shoulders appear broader and draw them back, expand your chest, improve your posture and strengthen your abdominals to reduce and prevent lower back pain. Perform these exercises three days a week, with a day of rest between days of exercise. Start off with a 2.5 kilogram hand weight and perform each exercise until you can complete three sets of 10 repetitions with ease. As you become stronger and more experienced, you can increase the load of the weights.

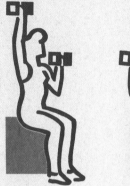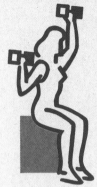

1. Strengthen your shoulders and upper arms by alternately raising and lowering dumbbells with your palms facing forwards.

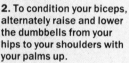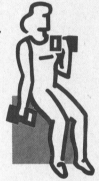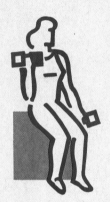

2. To condition your biceps, alternately raise and lower the dumbbells from your hips to your shoulders with your palms up.

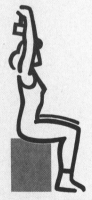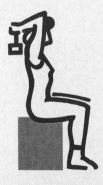

3. To condition the back of your upper arms and your upper back muscles, hold the upper end of a dumbbell with both hands over your head. Lower the weight behind your head, then raise it to the starting position.

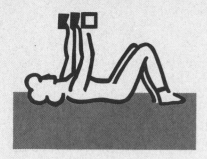 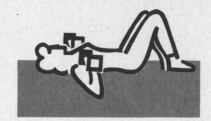

4. Lie on your back with your feet flat on an exercise bench. Face your palms forwards and raise the dumbbells directly over your shoulders. Lower the weights to slightly below your shoulders.

5. On an exercise bench, raise the dumbbells directly over your shoulders and keep your elbows slightly bent. Lower the dumbbells outwards, and then return to the starting position to strengthen the chest.

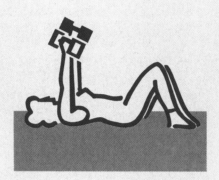 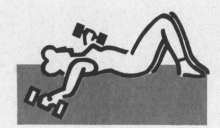

6. To condition your back and shoulder muscles, grasp two dumbbells and sit on a bench. Bend at the waist so that the dumbbells hang near the ankles. Slowly raise the dumbbells sideways to about shoulder level and then lower again. Do not attempt this exercise if you have any back problems.

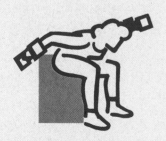

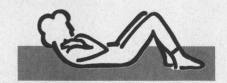

7. Perform bent-knee curls to strengthen the abdominals — you do not need to use dumbbells for this exercise. Lie on your back with your feet flat on the floor and your hands across your chest. Curl only your head and upper back off the floor and return to the starting position.

SOLE IN PARCHMENT ▼

White fish contains the same quality protein as red meat, but with a much lower calorie count. This cooking method keeps white fish moist.

CALORIES per serving	180
49% Carbohydrate	22 g
28% Protein	13 g
23% Fat	5 g
CALCIUM	40 mg
IRON	2 mg
SODIUM	255 mg

20 g (¾ oz) butter
45 g (1½ oz) spring onions, sliced
2 teaspoons lemon juice
1 garlic clove, crushed
½ teaspoon caraway seeds
¼ teaspoon salt
⅛ teaspoon paprika
Black pepper

Dash of Tabasco sauce
250 g (8 oz) sole fillets, cut into 4 equal pieces
6 small unpeeled red potatoes (about 400 g/14 oz), boiled and sliced 5 mm/¼ inch thick
175 g (6 oz) mange-tout, trimmed and blanched

Preheat the oven to 180°C (350°F or Mark 4). Melt the butter in a small saucepan over low heat. Stir in the spring onions, lemon juice, garlic, caraway seeds, salt, paprika, pepper and Tabasco sauce. Cook for 2 to 3 minutes, or until fragrant; set aside.

Cut out four 30 cm (12 inch) circles of baking parchment or aluminium foil. Place a portion of sole on one half of each circle and divide the potatoes and mange-tout among the four portions. Spoon the butter mixture over each portion, then fold the other half of the parchment over the fish and vegetables and firmly crimp the edges to seal them. Place the packets on a baking sheet and bake for 12 minutes, or until the fish flakes when tested with a knife. Place each packet on a plate and open just before serving.   Makes 4 servings

PASTA AND CAULIFLOWER WITH SESAME SAUCE

The vegetables here make for generous portions and provide twice your daily requirement of vitamin C while adding only 30 calories per serving.

400 g (14 oz) cauliflower florets
12.5 cl (4 fl oz) plain low-fat yogurt
4 teaspoons sesame oil
1 tablespoon toasted sesame seeds
1 teaspoon lemon juice

1 large sweet red pepper, cut into 5 mm (¼ inch) wide strips
250 g (8 oz) spinach fusilli (spiral pasta)
½ teaspoon salt
¼ teaspoon hot red pepper flakes
Black pepper

Bring a large saucepan of water to the boil. Add the cauliflower and cook for about 10 minutes, or until crisp but tender when pierced with a fork. Meanwhile, for the dressing, whisk together the yogurt, oil, sesame seeds and lemon juice in a large bowl. Add the pepper strips and toss to coat; set aside.

Reserving the boiling water, use a slotted spoon to transfer the cauliflower to a colander; cool under cold running water and drain. Cook the pasta in the boiling water for 8 minutes, or according to the packet directions until *al dente*; cool under cold water and drain thoroughly. Add the pasta and cauliflower to the dressing and toss until well combined. Add the salt and red pepper flakes, and black pepper to taste, and toss again.   Makes 4 servings

CALORIES per serving	320
60% Carbohydrate	49 g
15% Protein	12 g
25% Fat	9 g
CALCIUM	107 mg
IRON	3 mg
SODIUM	313 mg

Sole in Parchment ▷

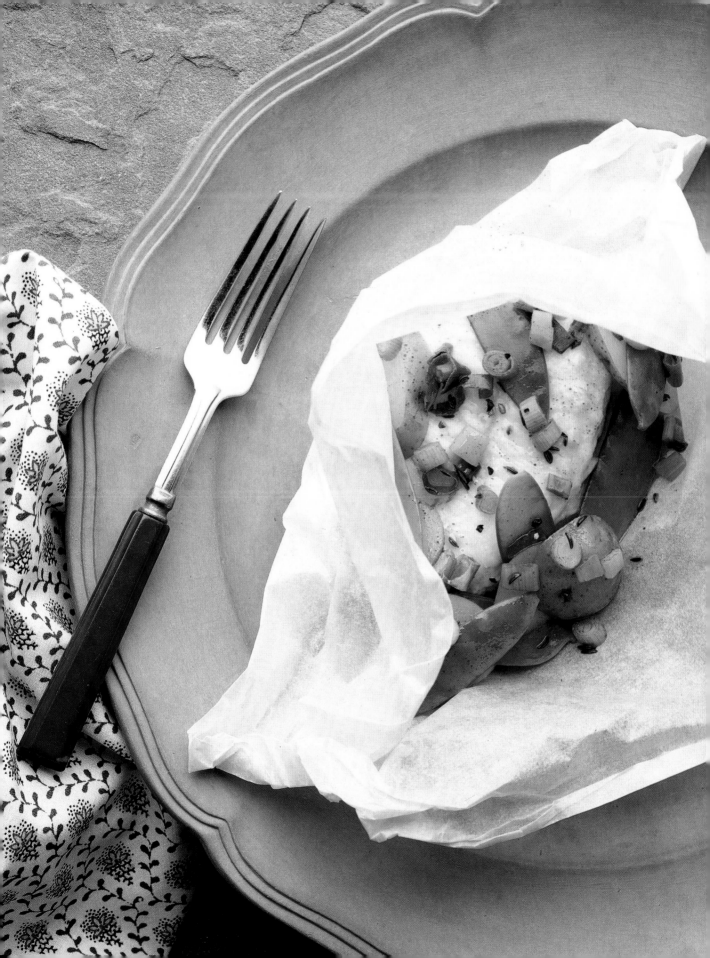

TOMATO AND BASIL FLAN WITH CHÈVRE ▼

The paper-thin pastry leaves called phyllo are usually brushed with melted butter before baking, but they work well here without the added fat.

CALORIES per serving	270
50% Carbohydrate	36 g
21% Protein	15 g
29% Fat	9 g
CALCIUM	155 mg
IRON	5 mg
SODIUM	392 mg

750 g (1½ lb) plum tomatoes
2 tablespoons low-sodium
   chicken stock
175 g (6 oz) onion, chopped
175 g (6 oz) spinach, chopped
250 g (8 oz) yellow or green
   courgettes, diced
90 g (3 oz) mushrooms, chopped
4 tablespoons chopped fresh
   basil

1 garlic clove, crushed
¼ teaspoon salt
¼ teaspoon pepper
4 sheets phyllo pastry
3 large eggs
4 tablespoons plain low-fat
   yogurt
Pinch of grated nutmeg
60 g (2 oz) chèvre (mild goat
   cheese), cut into small pieces

Preheat the oven to 180°C (350°F or Mark 4). Peel, seed and chop the tomatoes and set aside in a colander to drain. Heat the stock in a large non-stick frying pan over high heat. Add the onion, reduce the heat to medium and cook, stirring occasionally, for 5 minutes. Add the tomatoes, spinach, courgettes, mushrooms, basil, garlic, salt and pepper, and cover the pan. Cook, stirring occasionally, for another 5 minutes. Uncover the pan and cook, stirring, for 2 minutes more, or until the spinach is wilted. Remove the pan from the heat and set aside to cool.

Separate the phyllo. Fit one sheet into a 21 cm (8½ inch) flan tin, folding the edges to leave a 5 cm (2 inch) overhang. Repeat with the remaining phyllo. In a small bowl, whisk together the eggs, yogurt and nutmeg. Using a slotted spoon to drain the vegetables well, spoon them into the flan tin. Pour the egg mixture over the vegetables and dot with the chèvre. Roll and crimp the edges of the phyllo to form a rim and very lightly oil it. Bake the flan for 40 minutes, or until the filling is set and the pastry is light golden. Let the flan stand for 5 minutes, then cut it into quarters and serve.   Makes 4 servings

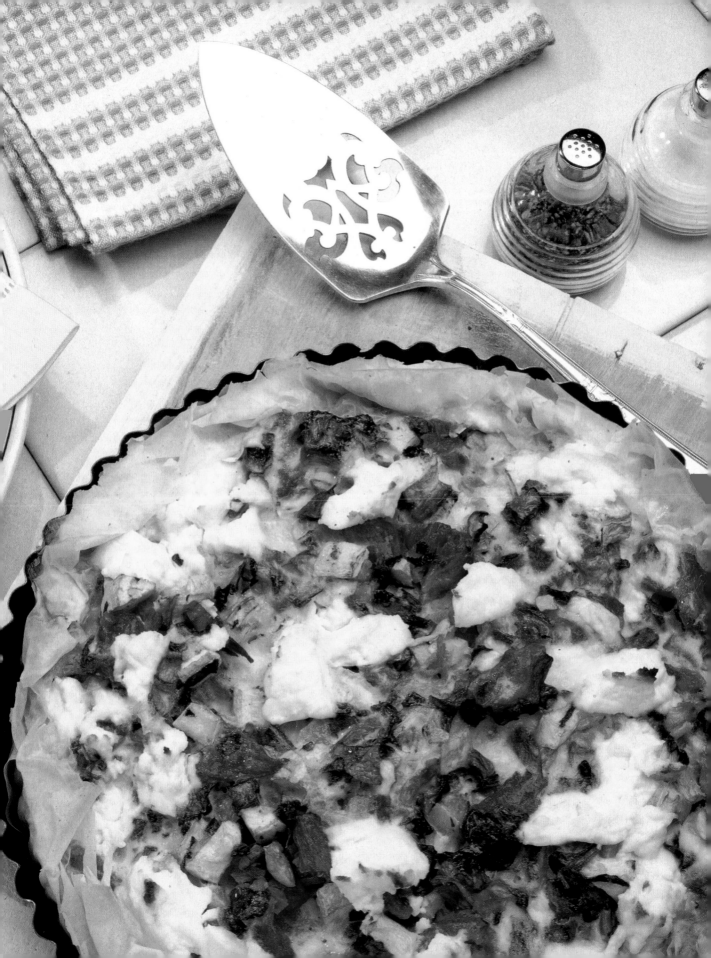

STRAWBERRY SHORTCAKE WITH YOGURT BISCUITS

A luxurious dessert does not have to be high in calories. Yogurt replaces some of the fat in these biscuits, and low-fat ricotta, instead of whipped cream, tops them.

300 g (10 oz) fresh strawberries	1 teaspoon baking powder
4 teaspoons brown sugar	¼ teaspoon bicarbonate of soda
60 g (2 oz) low-fat ricotta cheese	¼ teaspoon salt
1 tablespoon lemon juice	¼ teaspoon ground cinnamon
1½ teaspoons grated lemon rind	2½ tablespoons soft margarine,
175 g (6 oz) plain flour,	well chilled
approximately	4 tablespoons plain low-fat yogurt

Wash, hull and slice the strawberries and toss them with 2 teaspoons of the sugar in a small bowl. For the ricotta cream, mix together the ricotta, lemon juice, lemon rind and remaining sugar in another small bowl; set aside.

Preheat the oven to 230°C (450°F or Mark 8). Lightly grease a baking sheet. In a large bowl, stir together the flour, baking powder, bicarbonate of soda, salt and cinnamon. Using a pastry blender or two knives, cut in the margarine until the mixture resembles coarse crumbs. Add the yogurt and 4 tablespoons of cold water and stir briefly, then form the dough into a ball with your hands. On a lightly floured surface, knead the dough a few times then roll it out to a 1 cm (½ inch) thickness. Using a 6 cm (2½ inch) round cutter, cut out eight biscuits. Place them on the baking sheet and bake for 10 to 12 minutes, or until golden. Split the biscuits and place two of the bottom halves on each of four plates. Top each half with some of the strawberries and ricotta cream and cover with the biscuit tops.   Makes 4 servings

GRILLED VEGETABLE-CHEDDAR SANDWICH ▼

This sandwich is reminiscent of a cheeseburger — with less than half the fat.

75 g (6 oz) aubergine, cut into	100 g (3½ oz) spring onions,
5 mm (¼ inch) thick slices	thinly sliced
175 g (6 oz) mushrooms, sliced	250 g (8 oz) lettuce, torn into
125 g (4 oz) Cheddar cheese,	bite-sized pieces
grated	8 small slices wholemeal bread
200 g (7 oz) bean sprouts	2 tablespoons Dijon mustard

Preheat the oven to 180°C (350°F or Mark 4). Lightly oil a baking sheet, lay the aubergine slices on it and bake for 10 minutes, or until tender; set aside to cool. Meanwhile, place the mushrooms in a medium-sized frying pan with 2 tablespoons of water and cook over medium heat for 3 to 5 minutes, or until softened. Divide the cheese, mushrooms, bean sprouts, spring onions and lettuce among four of the slices of bread and top with the aubergine slices. Spread the remaining slices of bread with the mustard, place them on the sandwiches and press them firmly. Lightly oil a large non-stick frying pan and heat it over medium-high heat. Place the sandwiches cheese-side down in the pan and heat them, pressing with a metal spatula, for 3 to 4 minutes, or until the cheese is melted. Turn the sandwiches and cook for another 3 to 4 minutes, or until the bread is lightly browned.   Makes 4 servings

CALORIES per serving	270
65% Carbohydrate	43 g
11% Protein	7 g
24% Fat	7 g
CALCIUM	146 mg
IRON	2 mg
SODIUM	369 mg

H eading for the salad bar is a good lunchtime instinct if you are trying to lose weight, but choose carefully: dressings and sauces can sabotage a low-calorie meal. A 60 g (2 oz) portion of cooked macaroni has about 75 calories, but the same amount of macaroni salad may have over 200 calories. A 60 g (2 oz) serving of tuna canned in brine has 140 calories, while an equal amount of tuna salad with mayonnaise has 190 calories.

CALORIES per serving	225
55% Carbohydrate	33 g
20% Protein	12 g
25% Fat	7 g
CALCIUM	215 mg
IRON	4 mg
SODIUM	564 mg

GREEN SALAD WITH CHICKEN AND MANGOES

You can get half of your daily requirement of niacin from the chicken and mangoes in this salad.

250 g (8 oz) boneless skinless
    chicken breast
12.5 cl (4 fl oz) low-sodium
    chicken stock
4 tablespoons lemon juice
2 tablespoons olive oil
1 teaspoon finely chopped fresh
    tarragon, or ¼ teaspoon dried
    tarragon, crumbled
¼ teaspoon salt

¼ teaspoon black pepper
1 cos lettuce
2 bunches watercress
300 g (10 oz) sweet red peppers,
    diced
75 g (2½ oz) red cabbage,
    shredded
100 g (3½ oz) spring onions,
    finely chopped
4 mangoes, peeled and diced

CALORIES per serving	325
54% Carbohydrate	47 g
24% Protein	21 g
22% Fat	9 g
CALCIUM	241 mg
IRON	4 mg
SODIUM	236 mg

Place the chicken in a small saucepan, add cold water to cover and bring to the boil over medium-high heat. Reduce the heat so that the water simmers and poach the chicken for 5 minutes, or until cooked through; transfer it to a plate and set aside to cool to room temperature.

For the dressing, whisk together the stock, lemon juice, oil, tarragon, salt and pepper in a small bowl; set aside. Wash the lettuce and watercress. Tear the lettuce into bite-sized pieces, trim the watercress and combine the greens in a large bowl. Add the peppers, cabbage and spring onions and toss well.

Cut the chicken diagonally into thin slices. Whisk the dressing briefly to reblend it. Add the chicken, mangoes and dressing to the salad and toss gently. Divide the salad among four plates and serve.　　Makes 4 servings

Green Salad with Chicken and Mangoes

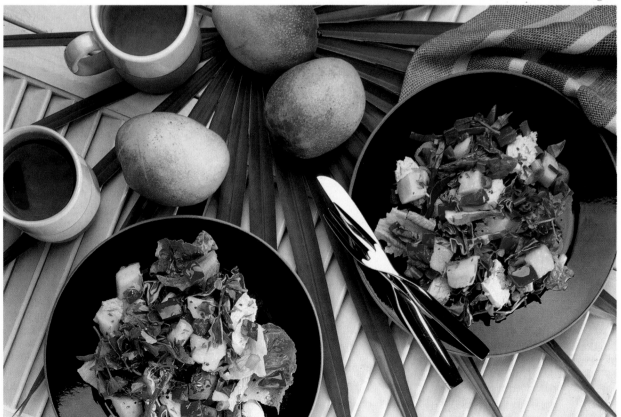

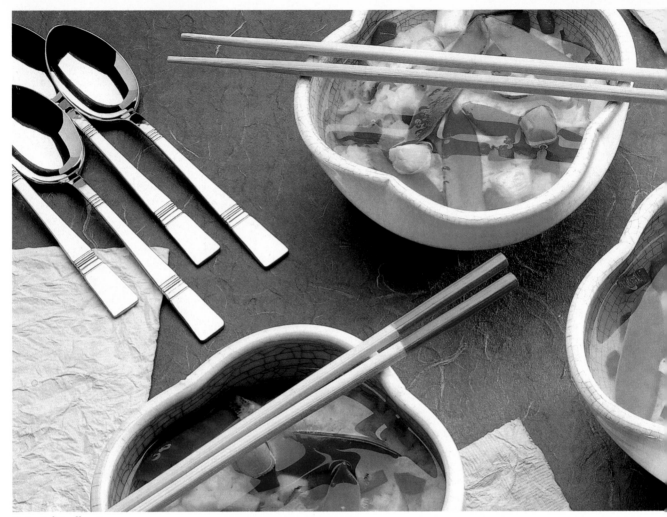

Oriental Scallop Soup

ORIENTAL SCALLOP SOUP ▼

Scallops are lower in fat and cholesterol than most fish and shellfish.

2 teaspoons vegetable oil	175 g (6 oz) carrots, chopped
60 g (2 oz) queen scallops	150 g (5 oz) fresh shiitake or
1 litre (1¾ pints) low-sodium	button mushrooms, sliced
chicken stock	125 g (4 oz) cooked white rice
45 g (1½ oz) spring onions,	75 g (2½ oz) sweet red pepper,
chopped	finely diced
1 teaspoon finely chopped fresh	90 g (3 oz) mange-tout, trimmed
ginger root	4 tablespoons sake

CALORIES per serving	140
59% Carbohydrate	20 g
23% Protein	7 g
18% Fat	3 g
CALCIUM	50 mg
IRON	3 mg
SODIUM	95 mg

Heat the oil in a medium-sized saucepan over medium heat. Add the scallops and sauté for 2 minutes, or until they are opaque and firm; transfer to a small bowl and set aside. Simmer the stock, spring onions, ginger and carrots in the saucepan, over medium heat, for 15 minutes. Strain the stock into a bowl and discard the solids. Return the stock to the pan, add the mushrooms and simmer for 2 minutes, or until the mushrooms are soft. Stir in the scallops, rice, red pepper, mange-tout, sake and 12.5 cl (4 fl oz) of water, and cook for another 3 minutes, or until the soup is heated through.   Makes 4 servings

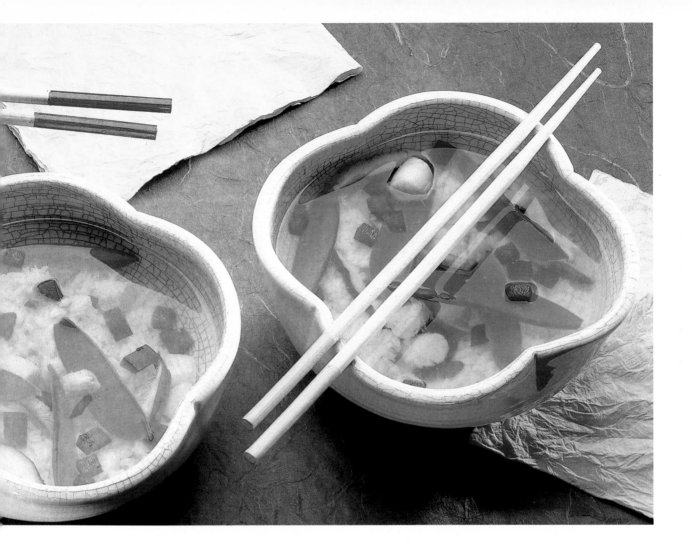

VELVETY VEGETABLE DRINK ▼

You can prepare this drink the day before serving it and chill it overnight.
With a salad and some wholemeal bread, it makes a light lunch.

50 cl (16 fl oz) low-sodium tomato juice	90 g (3 oz) celery, finely chopped
Small bunch fresh parsley	125 g (4 oz) sweet red pepper, finely chopped
10 watercress sprigs	4 tablespoons plain low-fat yogurt
125 g (4 oz) carrots, finely chopped	1 teaspoon olive oil, preferably extra-virgin

In a medium-sized saucepan, combine the tomato juice, parsley, watercress, carrots, celery and red pepper and bring to the boil over medium-high heat. Cover the pan, reduce the heat to low and simmer for 20 minutes, or until the vegetables are soft. Remove the pan from the heat and let the mixture cool slightly. Remove and discard the stems from the parsley and watercress and return the leaves to the saucepan. Process the mixture in a blender until puréed, then set aside to cool. Transfer the mixture to a jug, stir in the yogurt and oil, cover and refrigerate until chilled. Divide the drink between two tall ice-filled glasses and serve.   Makes 2 servings

CALORIES per serving	145
67% Carbohydrate	27 g
15% Protein	6 g
18% Fat	3 g
CALCIUM	200 mg
IRON	6 mg
SODIUM	137 mg

THREE-MELON SALAD WITH
RASPBERRY VINAIGRETTE ▼

CALORIES per serving	240
59% Carbohydrate	39 g
10% Protein	7 g
31% Fat	9 g
CALCIUM	51 mg
IRON	1 mg
SODIUM	357 mg

The dressing can make or break a low-calorie salad: the vinaigrette, ricotta cheese and pecans used here total under 100 calories per serving. A comparable amount of blue cheese dressing has more than 200 calories.

3 tablespoons raspberry vinegar, or to taste
1 tablespoon safflower oil
1 tablespoon lemon juice
½ teaspoon salt
600 g (1¼ lb) cantaloupe melon flesh, cut into chunks
500 g (1 lb) honeydew melon flesh, cut into chunks

600 g (1¼ lb) watermelon flesh, balled or cut into chunks
90 g (3 oz) low-fat ricotta cheese
30 g (1 oz) fresh mint leaves, chopped
4 large cos lettuce leaves, washed and trimmed
2 tablespoons coarsely chopped pecan nuts

For the dressing, whisk together the vinegar, oil, lemon juice and salt in a small bowl; set aside. Combine the melon chunks in a large bowl, add the dressing and toss gently. Cover the bowl and refrigerate for at least 1 hour. Just before serving, crumble the cheese into a small bowl, add the mint and mash with a fork to combine. Line a serving platter with the lettuce leaves and mound the melon on it. Sprinkle the cheese over the melon and scatter the pecan nuts on top.   Makes 4 servings

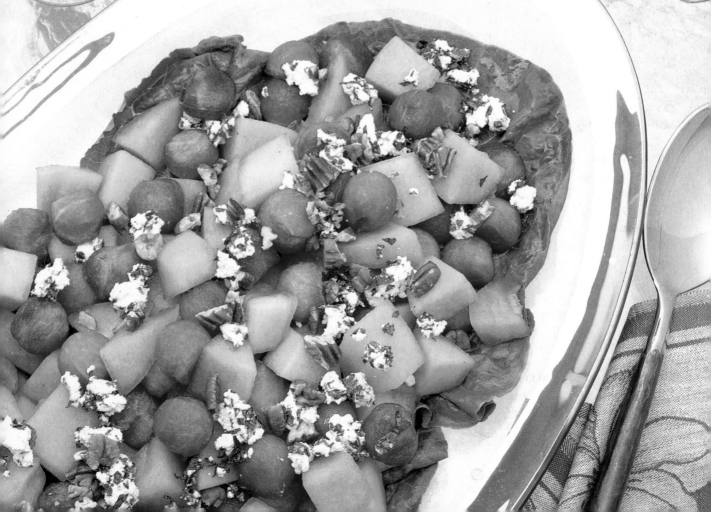

COUSCOUS

We in the West typically eat large portions of meat with small side dishes of vegetables and grains. This Moroccan-style meal, like many ethnic dishes, reverses those portions for a healthier, lower calorie lunch.

CALORIES per serving	375
65% Carbohydrate	53 g
14% Protein	12 g
21% Fat	8 g
CALCIUM	54 mg
IRON	2 mg
SODIUM	397 mg

2 tablespoons olive oil
½ teaspoon each ground
  cinnamon, cumin and paprika
2 or 3 saffron threads, crumbled
1 onion, sliced
90 g (3 oz) carrots, sliced
125 g (4 oz) parsnips, diced
10 dried apricot halves

1 small chicken thigh, skinned
225 g (7½ oz) canned plum
  tomatoes, drained and diced
250 g (8 oz) couscous
½ teaspoon salt
Black pepper to taste
2 tablespoons chopped
  fresh coriander

Heat the oil in a large heavy-bottomed saucepan over medium heat. Add the spices and saffron, and cook, stirring, for 2 minutes, or until fragrant. Add the onion, carrots, parsnips, apricots and chicken, and sauté, stirring occasionally, for 5 minutes. Add the tomatoes and 1.25 litres (2 pints) of water. Bring to the boil, reduce the heat to low, cover the pan and simmer for 30 minutes.

Remove the chicken from the pan, bone it and cut the meat into thin strips. Bring the mixture in the pan to the boil. Stir in the couscous using a wire whisk and cook for 30 seconds. Remove from the heat, cover and set aside for 7 minutes. When the couscous is ready, add the salt and pepper; scatter the chicken strips and coriander over it and serve.   Makes 4 servings

CURRIED VEGETABLE SOUP ▼

Puréed vegetables and semi-skimmed milk make this a creamy soup without cream.

2 tablespoons soft margarine
175 g (6 oz) onion, chopped
125 g (4 oz) carrots, diced
125 g (4 oz) celery, diced
1 garlic clove, crushed
1 tablespoon curry powder
850 g (28 oz) canned plum
  tomatoes
600 g (1¼ lb) cooked split
  peas (175 g/6 oz dried weight)

325 g (11 oz) sweetcorn kernels
½ teaspoon salt
½ teaspoon pepper
12.5 cl (4 fl oz) semi-skimmed
  milk
75 g (2½ oz) kale, shredded
4 tablespoons chopped fresh
  coriander
30 g (1 oz) savoury biscuits,
  preferably low-sodium

Melt the margarine in a large saucepan over medium heat. Add the onion, carrots, celery and garlic, and cook, stirring, for 5 minutes. Add the curry powder, the tomatoes and their liquid and 50 cl (16 fl oz) of water. Bring to the boil over medium-high heat, breaking up the tomatoes with the edge of a spoon. Reduce the heat to low and simmer the soup for 20 minutes. Add the split peas, sweetcorn, salt and pepper, and cook for 15 minutes. Using a slotted spoon, transfer three quarters of the vegetables to a food processor or blender and purée, then return the purée to the pan. Stir in the milk and cook until heated. Before serving, add the kale and stir until wilted. Sprinkle the soup with the coriander and serve with the biscuits.   Makes 4 servings

CALORIES per serving	265
64% Carbohydrate	45 g
18% Protein	12 g
18% Fat	6 g
CALCIUM	131 mg
IRON	4 mg
SODIUM	483 mg

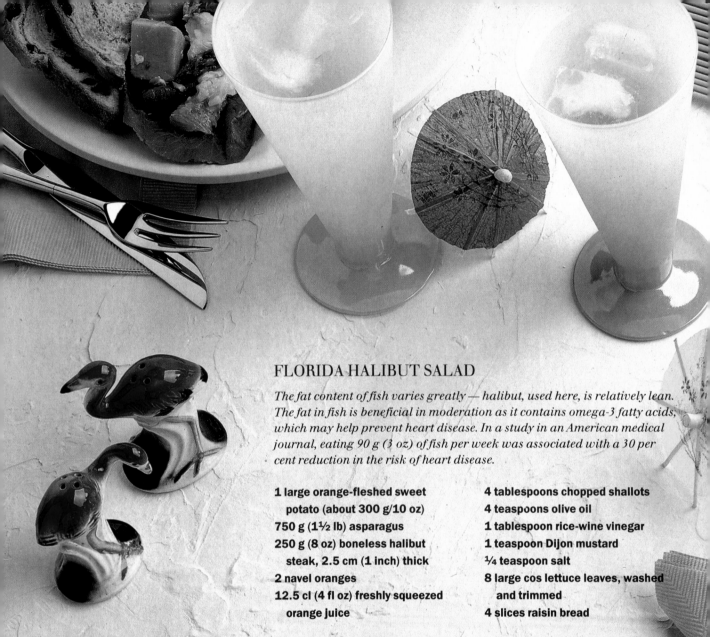

FLORIDA HALIBUT SALAD

The fat content of fish varies greatly — halibut, used here, is relatively lean. The fat in fish is beneficial in moderation as it contains omega-3 fatty acids, which may help prevent heart disease. In a study in an American medical journal, eating 90 g (3 oz) of fish per week was associated with a 30 per cent reduction in the risk of heart disease.

1 large orange-fleshed sweet potato (about 300 g/10 oz)	4 tablespoons chopped shallots
750 g (1½ lb) asparagus	4 teaspoons olive oil
250 g (8 oz) boneless halibut steak, 2.5 cm (1 inch) thick	1 tablespoon rice-wine vinegar
2 navel oranges	1 teaspoon Dijon mustard
12.5 cl (4 fl oz) freshly squeezed orange juice	¼ teaspoon salt
	8 large cos lettuce leaves, washed and trimmed
	4 slices raisin bread

Bring a small saucepan of water to the boil. Wash and trim the sweet potato; do not peel it. Cut the potato into 2.5 cm (1 inch) chunks and cook it for 20 minutes, or until it is tender. Meanwhile, bring a large pan of water to the boil. Trim the asparagus, cut it into 2.5 cm (1 inch) pieces and cook it for 5 to 7 minutes, or until it is tender but still crisp. Drain, cool under cold water and set aside to drain again. When the potato is done, drain and set aside to cool.

Preheat the oven to 180°C (350°F or Mark 4). Rinse and pat dry the halibut, place it in a small baking pan and bake it for 10 minutes, or until the fish flakes when tested with a fork; set aside to cool. Peel and segment the oranges and remove the membranes; set aside. For the dressing, stir together the orange juice, shallots, oil, vinegar, mustard and salt in a small bowl. In a large bowl, combine the potato, asparagus, halibut and oranges. Add the dressing and toss, breaking up the fish as little as possible. Cover and refrigerate the salad for 3 to 4 hours, tossing it twice while it is chilling.

To serve, line four plates with the lettuce and mound the halibut salad on top. Toast the bread and serve it with the salad.   Makes 4 servings

CALORIES per serving	305
57% Carbohydrate	45 g
24% Protein	19 g
19% Fat	7 g
CALCIUM	113 mg
IRON	3 mg
SODIUM	307 mg

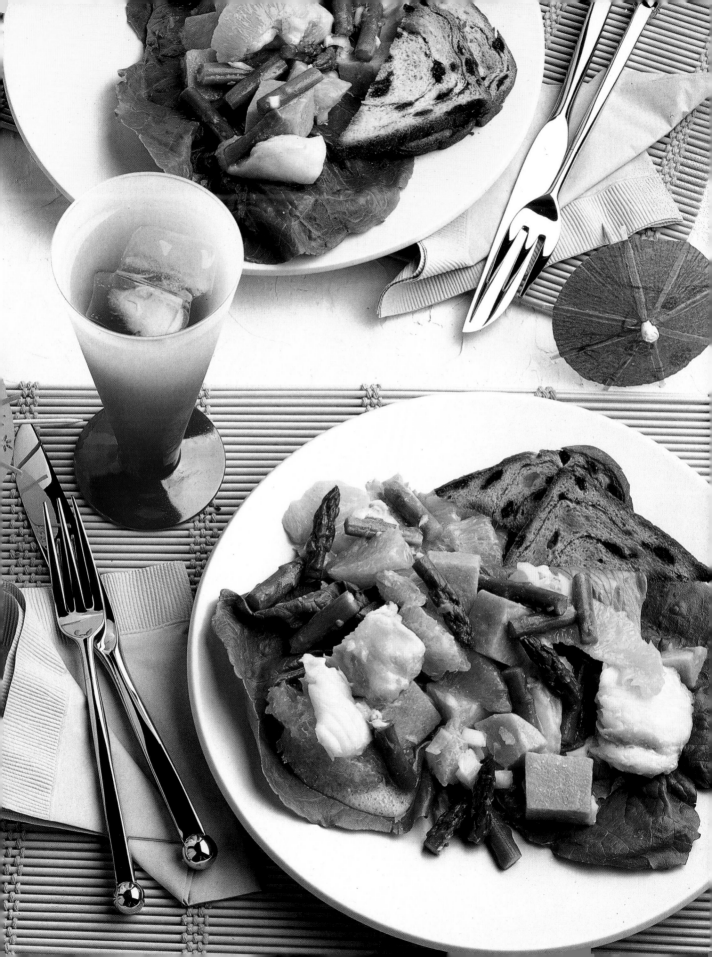

PRAWN MADRAS SANDWICH

Most shellfish is low in calories and rich in fluorine, a mineral that may help guard against calcium loss and osteoporosis.

CALORIES per serving	330
62% Carbohydrate	52 g
24% Protein	21 g
14% Fat	5 g
CALCIUM	130 mg
IRON	5 mg
SODIUM	727 mg

125 g (4 oz) yellow lentils
175 g (6 oz) onion, chopped
1 bay leaf
400 g (14 oz) canned chopped
  tomatoes, with their liquid
75 g (2½ oz) sweet green
  pepper, chopped
1 tablespoon olive oil
1 tablespoon crushed garlic
1 tablespoon finely chopped fresh
  ginger root

1½ teaspoons ground coriander
1 teaspoon ground turmeric
¾ teaspoon chili powder
125 g (4 oz) shelled raw prawns,
  cut in thirds
125 g (4 oz) frozen peas
¾ teaspoon salt
⅛ teaspoon Tabasco sauce, or
  to taste
Four 60 g (2 oz) pitta breads
4 tablespoons plain low-fat yogurt

Place the lentils in a medium-sized saucepan with 35 cl (12 fl oz) of water, the onion and bay leaf, and bring to the boil over medium-high heat. Cover the pan, reduce the heat to low and simmer for 30 minutes. Add the tomatoes and green pepper, and cook for 30 minutes, or until the lentils are tender.

Heat the oil in a medium-sized frying pan over medium heat. Add the garlic and ginger and sauté for 1 minute. Add the coriander, turmeric and chili powder, and cook for another minute. Reduce the heat to medium low, add the lentil mixture and cook for 5 minutes, or until thick. Add the prawns, peas, salt and Tabasco sauce, and cook for 5 minutes, or until the prawns are opaque.

Cut the pitta breads in half crosswise (warm them slightly if desired) and divide the lentil mixture among the halves. Spoon ½ tablespoon of yogurt into each pitta pocket and serve. *Makes 4 servings*

RASPBERRY FREEZE WITH LEMON SAUCE

Dieters need not give up dessert if they choose wisely. Instead of ice cream, made with egg yolks and double cream, have this freeze made with egg whites and semi-skimmed milk. This dessert is also a good source of vitamin C.

750 g (1½ lb) frozen
  unsweetened raspberries,
  partially thawed
12.5 cl (4 fl oz) apple juice
  concentrate
12.5 cl (4 fl oz) semi-skimmed
  milk
4 tablespoons evaporated
  skimmed milk

1½ teaspoons cornflour
2 teaspoons grated lemon rind
2 egg whites
2 tablespoons sugar
1 tablespoon lemon juice
2 tablespoons chopped fresh
  mint, plus 4 mint sprigs
  for garnish

A ttesting to the hunger-satisfying qualities of complex carbohydrates, a study at an American university showed that obese volunteers took in about 1,570 calories per day when the foods available were high in complex carbohydrates; when the foods were low in complex carbohydrates but high in fat, the volunteers consumed closer to 3,000 calories per day.

CALORIES per serving	205
83% Carbohydrate	45 g
10% Protein	6 g
7% Fat	2 g
CALCIUM	132 mg
IRON	1 mg
SODIUM	68 mg

For the raspberry freeze, place the raspberries and apple juice concentrate in a food processor or blender and process until puréed. Put the purée through a nylon sieve to remove the seeds, then transfer it to a freezer container and freeze it for at least 1 hour.

Meanwhile, make the sauce. In a medium-sized saucepan, stir together the

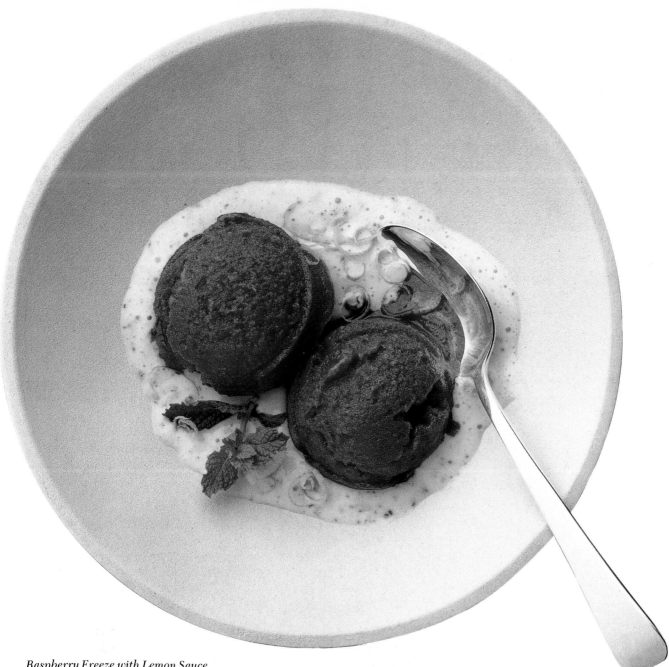

Raspberry Freeze with Lemon Sauce

semi-skimmed milk, evaporated milk and cornflour until smooth. Add 1 teaspoon of the lemon rind and bring the mixture to the boil over medium heat, stirring constantly; remove the pan from the heat and set aside. In a medium-sized bowl, whisk together the egg whites, sugar and lemon juice until frothy, then gradually whisk in the hot milk mixture. Return the mixture to the saucepan, add the mint and cook over low heat, stirring constantly, for 5 minutes, or until the sauce is thickened. Transfer the sauce to a small bowl, cover and refrigerate until well chilled.

To serve, let the raspberry mixture thaw at room temperature for 30 minutes, or until soft enough to scoop. Pour a quarter of the lemon sauce on to each of four dessert plates. Divide the raspberry freeze among the plates and garnish with the mint sprigs and remaining lemon rind.   Makes 4 servings

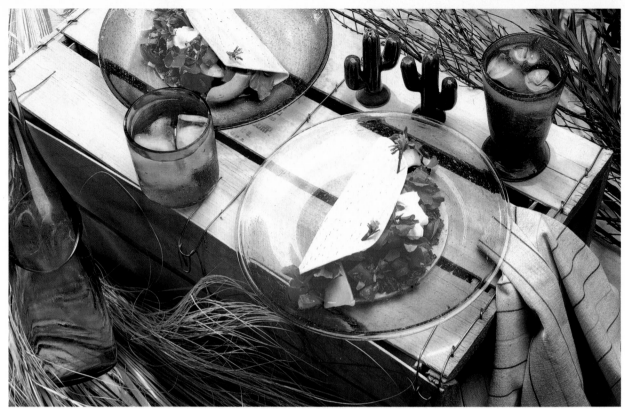

South of the Border Sandwiches

SOUTH OF THE BORDER SANDWICHES ▼

Beans, loaded with filling fibre, are usually cooked in lard and topped with soured cream in Mexican dishes. This recipe cuts the fat but not the flavour.

90 g (3 oz) dried black beans
1 large tomato, coarsely chopped
45 g (1½ oz) onion, chopped
1 tablespoon chopped fresh
   coriander
2 teaspoons balsamic vinegar,
   or to taste

4 flour tortillas (recipe page 52)
½ avocado
⅛ teaspoon salt
Pepper
75 g (2½ oz) watercress, washed
   and trimmed
4 tablespoons plain low-fat yogurt

Place the beans in a medium-sized saucepan with cold water to cover. Cover the pan and leave the beans to soak for 8 hours, or overnight.

Drain the beans, add 1.25 litres (2 pints) of fresh water and bring to the boil. Boil for 10 minutes, then reduce the heat and simmer for 1 hour, or until the beans are soft. Drain, reserving 1 tablespoon of liquid; set aside to cool.

Preheat the oven to 180°C (350°F or Mark 4). To make a salsa, stir the tomato, onion, coriander and vinegar together in a small bowl; set aside. Wrap the tortillas in foil and heat them in the oven for 5 minutes. Meanwhile, peel the avocado half and cut it into thin slices. Using a fork or potato masher, coarsely mash the beans, adding some of the cooking liquid if they are very dry. Stir in the salt and add pepper to taste.

Place each tortilla on a plate. Spread one half of each tortilla with a quarter of the beans, then divide the salsa, avocado slices, watercress and yogurt among them. Fold the tortillas over the filling and serve.　　Makes 4 servings

CALORIES per serving	240
61% Carbohydrate	38 g
16% Protein	10 g
23% Fat	6 g
CALCIUM	123 mg
IRON	4 mg
SODIUM	94 mg

96

ROASTED RED PEPPER SOUP WITH CROUTONS ▼

A recent study showed that dieters who had low-fat soups at least four times a week lost more weight than those who had soup less often.

CALORIES per serving	140
56% Carbohydrate	21 g
12% Protein	5 g
32% Fat	5 g
CALCIUM	99 mg
IRON	2 mg
SODIUM	360 mg

4 large sweet red peppers
1 small potato, boiled, peeled and quartered
125 g (4 oz) carrots, grated
25 cl (8 fl oz) low-sodium chicken stock
25 cl (8 fl oz) semi-skimmed milk

¼ teaspoon salt
¼ teaspoon pepper
Three 1 cm (½ inch) thick slices French bread (about 30 g/1 oz)
1 tablespoon olive oil
2 garlic cloves, crushed

Preheat the grill. Pierce the red peppers in several places with a fork, then grill them 15 cm (6 inches) from the heat, turning frequently, for 20 minutes, or until well charred. Place the peppers in a paper bag and let them steam for 15 minutes. Peel, seed and quarter the peppers and place them in a food processor with the potato, half the carrots, the stock, milk, salt and pepper. Purée until smooth, then transfer to a medium-sized saucepan and set aside.

Cut the bread into 1 cm (½ inch) cubes, place them in a non-stick frying pan with the oil and garlic and sauté over medium-high heat for 5 minutes, or until the croutons are crisp. Remove the pan from the heat. Heat the soup over medium heat for 5 minutes, ladle it into four bowls and garnish with the croutons and the remaining carrots.   Makes 4 servings

Y *ou satisfy your appetite better when you eat whole fruits, such as oranges, apples and prunes, than when you drink their juices. The activity of chewing and the stomach-filling fibre in the fruit both contribute to this effect.*

TROPICAL BEAN SALAD

Adding a small amount of turkey (a complete protein) to this salad allows the body to make better use of the incomplete vegetable protein in the beans.

4 tablespoons low-sodium chicken stock
2 tablespoons Dijon mustard
2 tablespoons lemon juice
4 teaspoons olive oil
1 garlic clove, finely chopped
Black pepper to taste
3 tablespoons finely chopped fresh basil
1 large cos lettuce, washed

600 g (1¼ lb) cooked haricot beans (300 g/10 oz dried weight)
450 g (15 oz) fresh pineapple chunks
1 red onion, thinly sliced
6 plum tomatoes, cut into wedges
325 g (11 oz) seedless grapes
60 g (2 oz) smoked turkey, cut into chunks
12 blanched almonds, toasted

For the dressing, whisk together the stock, mustard, lemon juice, oil, garlic and pepper in a small bowl. Stir in the basil; set aside. Trim the lettuce and cut the leaves in half crosswise; wrap the top halves in plastic film and refrigerate. Cut the bottom halves into very thin strips, place them in a large serving bowl, add the beans, pineapple, onion, tomatoes, grapes and turkey and toss to combine. Add the dressing and toss again. Cover and refrigerate for 3 hours, or until the salad is chilled and the flavours blended.

To serve, arrange the reserved lettuce leaves round the edges of the salad. Scatter the almonds over the salad and serve.   Makes 6 servings

CALORIES per serving	380
63% Carbohydrate	63 g
18% Protein	18 g
19% Fat	8 g
CALCIUM	112 mg
IRON	7 mg
SODIUM	257 mg

VEGETABLE, CHICKEN AND CHEESE MELT

If you replace a thick slice of cheese on a toasted sandwich with grated cheese, you can use much less. It melts faster, too.

CALORIES per serving	305
56% Carbohydrate	44 g
23% Protein	18 g
21% Fat	7 g
CALCIUM	168 mg
IRON	3 mg
SODIUM	464 mg

1 tablespoon olive oil
175 g (6 oz) onion, chopped
2 garlic cloves, crushed
3 sweet red peppers, coarsely diced
2 courgettes, sliced 5 mm (¼ inch) thick
Black pepper

125 g (4 oz) boned skinned chicken breast, cut into 1 cm (½ inch) chunks
Four 60 g (2 oz) wholemeal pitta breads
60 g (2 oz) low-fat mozzarella cheese, grated
175 g (6 oz) watercress leaves, washed

Heat 2½ teaspoons of the oil in a medium-sized non-stick frying pan over medium heat. Add the onion and garlic, and cook, stirring, for 4 minutes. Increase the heat to medium high, add the red peppers and courgettes, and cook, stirring, for 5 minutes. Add 12.5 cl (4 fl oz) of water and cook for 3 minutes more. Add pepper to taste and, using a slotted spoon, transfer the vegetables to a bowl to cool. Add the chicken to the pan and cook, stirring, over medium heat for 5 minutes or until cooked through. Transfer the chicken to a small bowl. Wipe the pan with paper towels; set aside.

Split the pitta breads and sprinkle the bottom halves with the mozzarella. Divide the vegetable mixture, chicken and watercress among the sandwiches and cover with the top halves of the pitta breads. Heat the remaining oil in the frying pan over medium-high heat. Place one sandwich at a time in the pan and heat it for 3 minutes, or until the cheese melts, then carefully turn and heat it for 2 minutes more.   Makes 4 servings

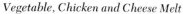

Vegetable, Chicken and Cheese Melt

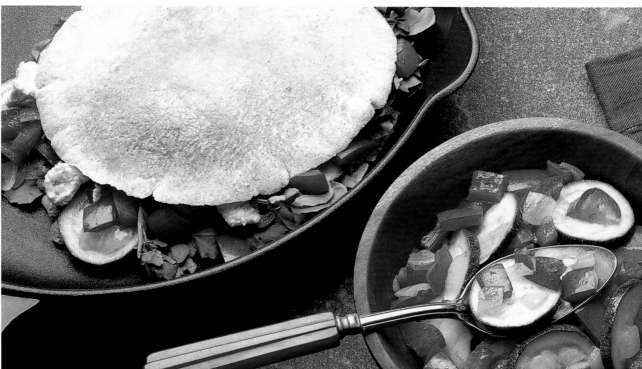

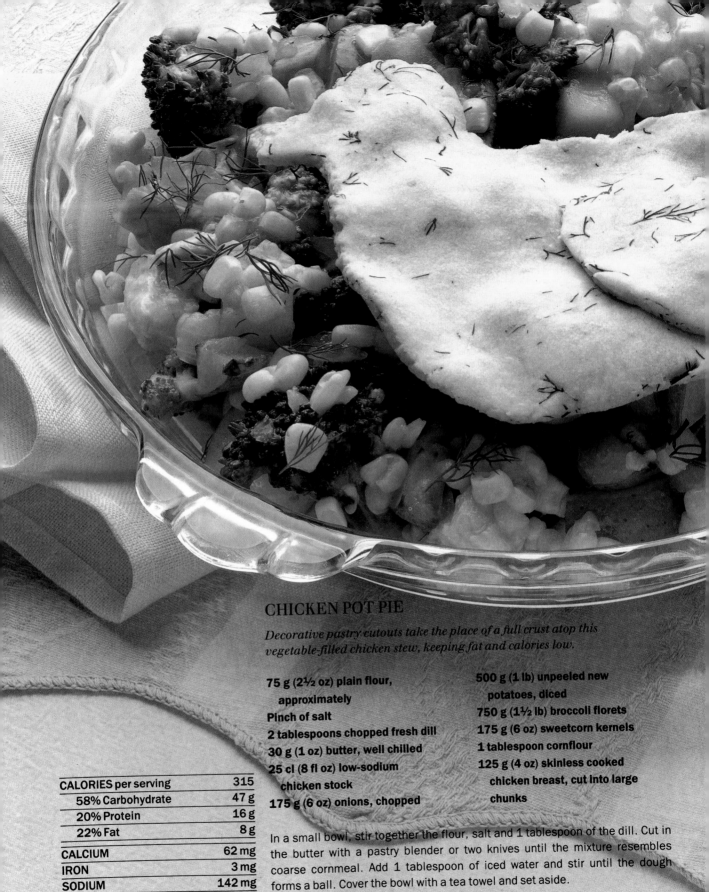

CHICKEN POT PIE

Decorative pastry cutouts take the place of a full crust atop this vegetable-filled chicken stew, keeping fat and calories low.

75 g (2½ oz) plain flour, approximately

Pinch of salt

2 tablespoons chopped fresh dill

30 g (1 oz) butter, well chilled

25 cl (8 fl oz) low-sodium chicken stock

175 g (6 oz) onions, chopped

500 g (1 lb) unpeeled new potatoes, diced

750 g (1½ lb) broccoli florets

175 g (6 oz) sweetcorn kernels

1 tablespoon cornflour

125 g (4 oz) skinless cooked chicken breast, cut into large chunks

CALORIES per serving	315
58% Carbohydrate	47 g
20% Protein	16 g
22% Fat	8 g
CALCIUM	62 mg
IRON	3 mg
SODIUM	142 mg

In a small bowl, stir together the flour, salt and 1 tablespoon of the dill. Cut in the butter with a pastry blender or two knives until the mixture resembles coarse cornmeal. Add 1 tablespoon of iced water and stir until the dough forms a ball. Cover the bowl with a tea towel and set aside.

INDEX

ACKNOWLEDGEMENTS

The tables on page 25 are reprinted courtesy of the Health Education Authority, United Kingdom.

The editors wish to thank Irena Hoare and Norma MacMillan.

Index prepared by Ian Tucker.

PHOTOGRAPHY CREDITS

Cover, page 3 and page 6: Julian Bajzert, London; all other photographs: Steven Mays, Rebus, Inc.

ILLUSTRATION CREDITS

Page 8, illustration: Tammi Colichio; page 11, illustration: Tammi Colichio; page 12, illustration: David Flaherty; page 15, illustration: David Flaherty; page 16, illustration: Tammi Colichio; page 18, illustration: David Flaherty; page 21, illustration: Tammi Colichio; page 26, illustration: Tammi Colichio; page 31, illustration: Brian Sisco; pages 34-35, chart: Brian Sisco; pages 36-37, chart: Brian Sisco; page 39, chart: Brian Sisco; page 41, chart: Brian Sisco; page 47, chart: Brian Sisco; pages 48-49, illustration: David Flaherty; page 79, chart: Brian Sisco; pages 80-81, illustration: David Flaherty; page 113, chart: Brian Sisco; page 115, illustration: Tammi Colichio.

Typeset by A.J. Latham Limited,
Dunstable, Bedfordshire, England
Printed by GEA, Milan and bound by GEP,
Cremona, Italy

lemon juice in a bowl. For the dressing, combine in a small bowl the quark, milk, chutney, curry powder, the remaining salt and 1 tablespoon of the lemon juice from the pears. In a large bowl, combine the rice and pasta with the red peppers, carrots, spring onions, pears and the drained currants. Add the dressing and toss well, then cover and refrigerate until well chilled.

To serve, line four plates with the lettuce and mound the salad on top. Sprinkle the salad with the pistachio nuts and serve.   Makes 4 servings

SCALLOP BISQUE

This soup has more potassium than two bananas, more vitamin C than two oranges, more calcium than a glass of whole milk and more iron than a glass of prune juice.

CALORIES per serving	325
47% Carbohydrate	39 g
22% Protein	18 g
31% Fat	11 g
CALCIUM	350 mg
IRON	4 mg
SODIUM	498 mg

1 tablespoon vegetable oil
3 tablespoons plain flour
4 tablespoons finely chopped shallots
50 cl (16 fl oz) skimmed milk
12.5 cl (4 fl oz) low-sodium chicken stock
125 g (4 oz) carrots, grated
150 g (5 oz) sweet red pepper, diced

150 g (5 oz) sweet yellow pepper, diced
90 g (3 oz) mushrooms, sliced
60 g (2 oz) queen scallops
2 tablespoons quark
1½ teaspoons grated lemon rind
¼ teaspoon salt
Black pepper
2 tablespoons chopped parsley

Heat the oil in a large saucepan over medium heat. Add the flour and shallots, and cook, stirring, for 2 minutes. Do not let the flour brown. Whisk in the milk, stock and 12.5 cl (4 fl oz) of water and continue whisking until smooth. Add the carrots, sweet peppers and mushrooms and bring the mixture to the boil, then reduce the heat to low and simmer the soup for 15 minutes, or until the vegetables are tender. Transfer the soup to a food processor or blender and process until puréed. Return the soup to the saucepan, add the scallops and cook over medium-low heat for 5 minutes, or until the scallops are opaque. Stir in the quark, lemon rind, salt, and pepper to taste, and ladle the soup into two bowls. Sprinkle with the parsley and serve.   Makes 2 servings

GINGERED SQUASH AND CABBAGE

The appetizing contrast of crisp Chinese cabbage and creamy squash in this side dish can enliven a simple low-fat meal.

1 butternut squash
3 garlic cloves
25 cl (8 fl oz) low-sodium chicken stock
3 thick slices fresh ginger root

175 g (6 oz) Chinese cabbage, cut into 5 mm (¼ inch) wide strips
125 g (4 oz) fresh shiitake mushrooms, trimmed and sliced

CALORIES per serving	50
60% Carbohydrate	8 g
26% Protein	3 g
14% Fat	1 g
CALCIUM	58 mg
IRON	4 mg
SODIUM	15 mg

Peel and seed the squash and cut it into 5 mm (¼ inch) slices. Lightly crush the garlic. Bring the stock to the boil in a medium-sized pan over medium heat. Add the garlic and ginger, reduce the heat to low, cover and simmer for 10 minutes. Remove and discard the garlic and ginger. Add the cabbage, squash and mushrooms, cover the pan and simmer, stirring occasionally, for 10 minutes, or until the vegetables are tender.   Makes 4 servings

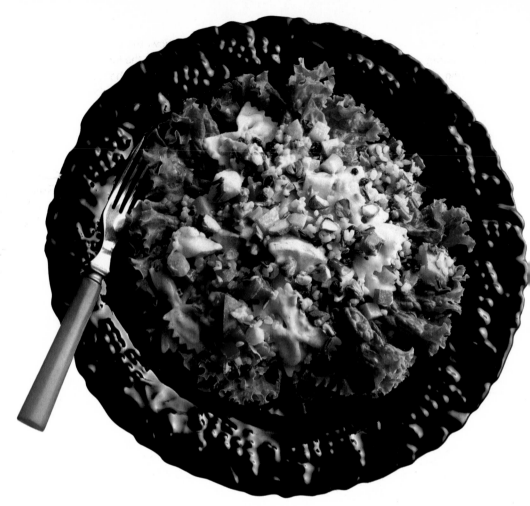

Two-Rice and Pasta Salad

TWO-RICE AND PASTA SALAD

Grains, pasta, fruit and nuts make this a satisfying main-dish salad.

CALORIES per serving	365
77% Carbohydrate	73 g
11% Protein	10 g
12% Fat	5 g
CALCIUM	115 mg
IRON	4 mg
SODIUM	474 mg

2 tablespoons currants
¾ teaspoon salt
75 g (2 ½ oz) wild rice
90 g (3 oz) brown rice
50 g (1¾ oz) small bow-tie pasta
350 g (12 oz) Anjou or Conference pears
2 tablespoons lemon Juice
4 tablespoons quark
4 tablespoons semi-skimmed milk

2 tablespoons chutney
2 teaspoons curry powder
150 g (5 oz) sweet red peppers, diced
125 g (4 oz) carrots, diced
60 g (2 oz) spring onions, chopped
8 large lettuce leaves
25 g (¾ oz) shelled toasted pistachio nuts

Place the currants in a small bowl with hot water to cover; set aside. Bring 2 litres (3½ pints) of water to the boil in a large saucepan over medium-high heat. Add ¼ teaspoon of the salt and the rices, and cook, stirring occasionally, for 40 minutes. Add the pasta and cook for 8 minutes. Drain the rice and pasta in a large strainer, cool under cold water and set aside to drain.

Core the pears, cut them into 2 cm (¾ inch) cubes and toss them with the

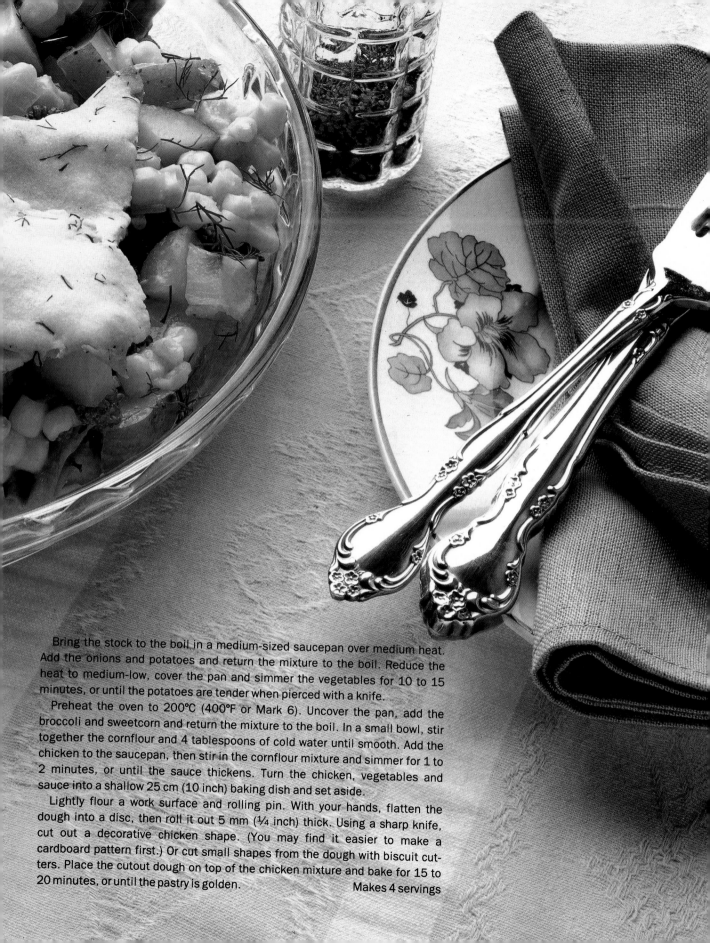

Bring the stock to the boil in a medium-sized saucepan over medium heat. Add the onions and potatoes and return the mixture to the boil. Reduce the heat to medium-low, cover the pan and simmer the vegetables for 10 to 15 minutes, or until the potatoes are tender when pierced with a knife.

Preheat the oven to 200°C (400°F or Mark 6). Uncover the pan, add the broccoli and sweetcorn and return the mixture to the boil. In a small bowl, stir together the cornflour and 4 tablespoons of cold water until smooth. Add the chicken to the saucepan, then stir in the cornflour mixture and simmer for 1 to 2 minutes, or until the sauce thickens. Turn the chicken, vegetables and sauce into a shallow 25 cm (10 inch) baking dish and set aside.

Lightly flour a work surface and rolling pin. With your hands, flatten the dough into a disc, then roll it out 5 mm (¼ inch) thick. Using a sharp knife, cut out a decorative chicken shape. (You may find it easier to make a cardboard pattern first.) Or cut small shapes from the dough with biscuit cutters. Place the cutout dough on top of the chicken mixture and bake for 15 to 20 minutes, or until the pastry is golden.

Makes 4 servings

APPLE, FENNEL AND PASTA SALAD

This salad gives you more than 12 grams of dietary fibre, 40 per cent of the daily amount recommended by the National Advisory Committee on Nutrition Education in the United Kingdom.

CALORIES per serving	380
63% Carbohydrate	62 g
15% Protein	14 g
22% Fat	10 g
CALCIUM	241 mg
IRON	3 mg
SODIUM	576 mg

150 g (5 oz) elbow macaroni

250 g (8 oz) frozen broad beans

4 tablespoons balsamic vinegar

1½ tablespoons olive oil

1 tablespoon apple juice concentrate

2 teaspoons chopped fresh oregano, or ¾ teaspoon dried oregano

½ teaspoon salt

¼ teaspoon pepper

3 red-skinned apples (about 500 g/1 lb)

2 tablespoons lemon juice

250 g (8 oz) bulb fennel, trimmed and thinly sliced

75 g (2½ oz) radishes, thinly sliced

45 g (1½ oz) Parmesan cheese

½ small head Batavian endive

Bring a large saucepan of water to the boil. Add the macaroni and cook for 8 minutes, or according to the packet directions until *al dente*; drain, rinse under cold water and set aside to drain thoroughly. Cook the broad beans according to the packet directions; drain and set aside.

For the dressing, whisk together the vinegar, oil, apple juice concentrate, oregano, salt and pepper; set aside. Core but do not peel the apples, then dice them and toss them with the lemon juice in a large bowl. Add the fennel, macaroni, broad beans, radishes and dressing, and toss well. Using a vegetable peeler or a sharp knife, cut the Parmesan into thin shavings; set aside.

To serve, wash and trim the Batavian endive. Line a platter with the leaves and mound the apple mixture on top. Scatter the Parmesan shavings over the salad and serve.

Makes 4 servings

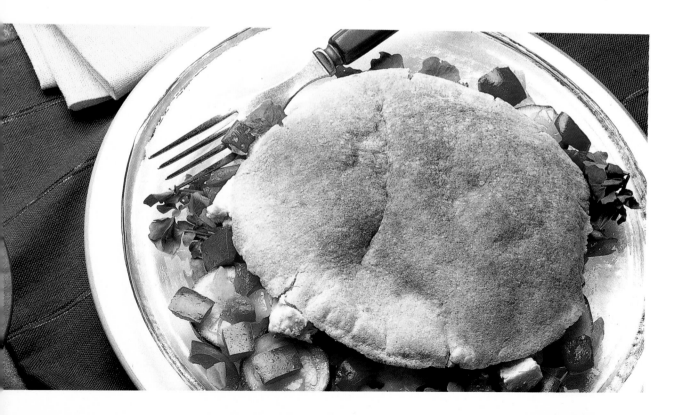

LIME BAVARIAN

CALORIES per serving	140
65% Carbohydrate	24 g
15% Protein	6 g
20% Fat	3 g
CALCIUM	78 mg
IRON	1 mg
SODIUM	93 mg

Using cream instead of skimmed milk would add 125 calories a serving.

1½ teaspoons gelatine	2 large eggs, separated
4 tablespoons freshly squeezed lime juice	4 tablespoons sugar
	Pinch of salt
17.5 cl (6 fl oz) skimmed milk	Pinch of cream of tartar
1½ teaspoons grated lime rind	225 g (7½ oz) fresh blueberries

Sprinkle the gelatine over the lime juice; set aside to soften. Bring the milk and lime rind to the boil in a heavy-bottomed saucepan then set aside to cool.

Using an electric mixer, beat the egg yolks with 3 tablespoons of the sugar in a medium-sized bowl until thick and pale. Whisk in the milk, return the mixture to the saucepan and cook over medium-low heat, stirring constantly, for 5 minutes, or until it coats the back of a spoon. Strain the mixture into the bowl, then add the gelatine mixture and stir until the gelatine is dissolved. Refrigerate, stirring occasionally, for 1 hour, or until it begins to thicken.

In a large bowl, beat the egg whites, salt and cream of tartar until frothy. Gradually beat in the remaining sugar and beat until soft peaks form. Fold the whites into the gelatine mixture. Spoon into four dessert bowls, cover and refrigerate for 4 hours. Serve topped with the blueberries.   Makes 4 servings

Colour can be a helpful guide to vitamin content when you choose fruits and vegetables. Generally, the deeper the colour, the higher the nutrient content. For example, apricots have more vitamin A than peaches, and oranges have more vitamin C and potassium than grapefruits. Acorn squash has more calcium and iron than crookneck squash, and kale is richer than lettuce in all nutrients.

SCALLOP AND ORANGE SALAD

Dark brown unhusked burghul is a very nutritious form of wheat.

2 navel oranges	¼ teaspoon salt
33 cl (11 fl oz) orange juice	¼ teaspoon pepper
175 g (6 oz) queen scallops	300 g (10 oz) sweet red pepper, diced
2 tablespoons finely chopped fresh ginger root	75 g (2½ oz) spring onions, sliced
1 tablespoon honey	175 g (6 oz) burghul
1 garlic clove, finely chopped	150 g (5 oz) lettuce leaves
4 tablespoons white wine vinegar	500 g (1 lb) broccoli florets, blanched
2 tablespoons olive oil	

Grate 2 teaspoons of orange rind; set aside. Peel and segment the oranges. Heat the orange juice in a large frying pan over medium-high heat, add the scallops and cook for 30 seconds; drain in a strainer set over a bowl. Return the orange juice to the pan, add the ginger, honey and garlic, and bring to the boil. Reduce the heat and cook, stirring occasionally, for 20 minutes, or until the liquid is reduced to about 12.5 cl (4 fl oz). Strain and set aside to cool.

In a large bowl, whisk together the vinegar, oil, salt and pepper. Stir in the scallops, orange liquid and segments, half the orange rind, the red pepper and half the spring onions; cover and refrigerate for 1 hour. Meanwhile, place the burghul in a medium-sized bowl and add 50 cl (16 fl oz) of cold water; set aside for 30 minutes, then drain and squeeze as dry as possible.

Line four plates with lettuce and top with the burghul. Arrange the scallops, broccoli and oranges on top. Dribble the dressing over the salads and sprinkle with the remaining spring onions and orange rind.   Makes 4 servings

CALORIES per serving	390
65% Carbohydrate	67 g
16% Protein	16 g
19% Fat	9 g
CALCIUM	126 mg
IRON	5 mg
SODIUM	228 mg

Scallop and Orange Salad ▷

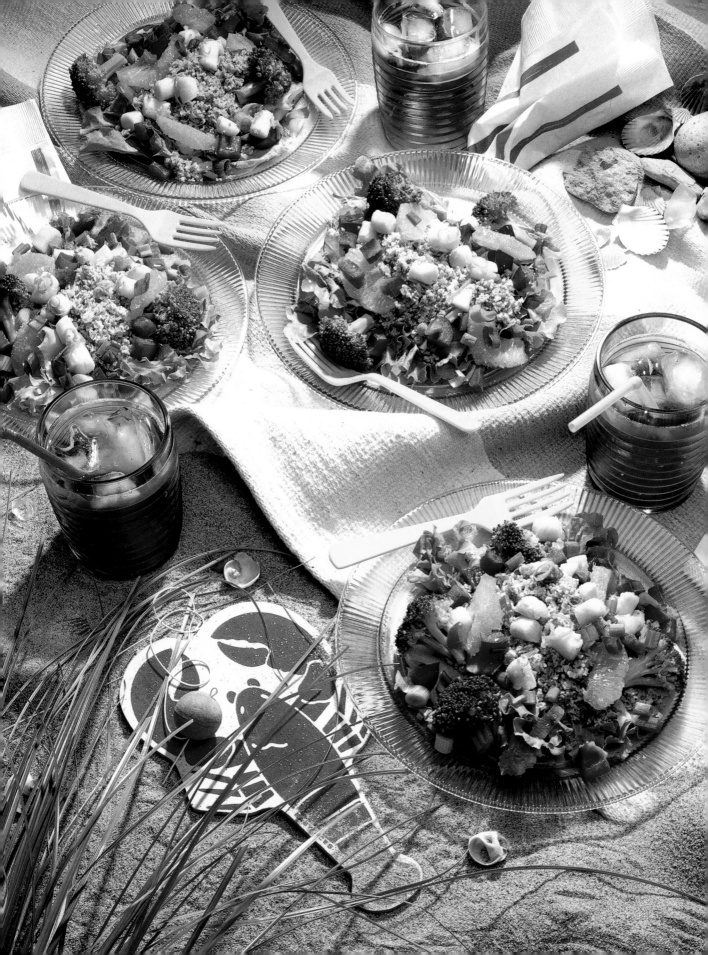

Mid-Afternoon Snacks

AUBERGINE CAVIARE

Unlike most aubergine spreads, this one contains just a teaspoon of oil.

CALORIES per serving	145
69% Carbohydrate	27 g
14% Protein	6 g
17% Fat	3 g
CALCIUM	109 mg
IRON	2 mg
SODIUM	267 mg

1.1 kg (2¼ lb) aubergines
1 sweet red pepper
1 onion
1 garlic clove
1 tablespoon toasted sesame
   seeds

1 tablespoon chopped parsley
1 teaspoon olive oil
1 teaspoon lemon juice
¼ teaspoon salt
Black pepper
4 slices wholemeal bread

Preheat the oven to 190°C (375°F or Mark 5). Prick the aubergines and red pepper with a fork, place them on a baking sheet with the unpeeled onion and bake for 45 minutes, or until the aubergines collapse and the onion is tender when pierced with a fork; set aside to cool.

Halve the aubergines and scoop the flesh into a food processor or blender. Halve, stem and seed the pepper, and peel the onion and garlic. Add them to the aubergines. Process the mixture, pulsing the machine on and off, just until very coarsely chopped. Transfer the mixture to a bowl and stir in the sesame seeds, parsley, oil, lemon juice, salt, and black pepper to taste. Cover and refrigerate the caviare for at least 1 hour. To serve, toast the bread, cut the slices into quarters and spread with the caviare.   Makes 4 servings

Chewy Citrus Thins

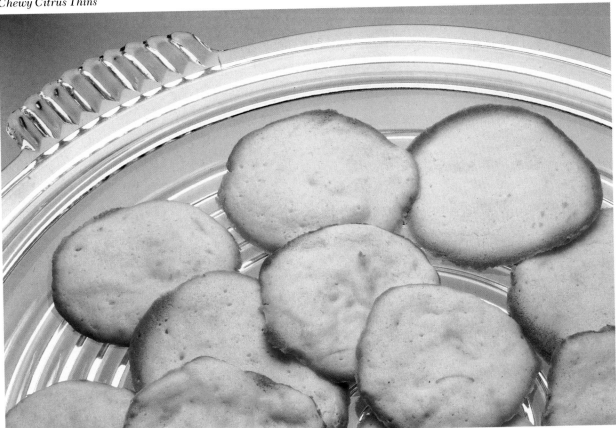

COURGETTE-RAISIN MUFFINS

Using courgettes in these muffins increases their fibre content, while adding a negligible number of calories.

75 g (2½ oz) rolled oats

15 g (½ oz) bran cereal

35 cl (12 fl oz) buttermilk

30 g (1 oz) margarine

2 tablespoons light brown sugar

1 large egg, lightly beaten

125 g (4 oz) wholemeal flour

1 teaspoon baking powder

1 teaspoon bicarbonate of soda

¼ teaspoon salt

¼ teaspoon ground cinnamon

150 g (5 oz) courgettes, grated and squeezed dry

75 g (2½ oz) raisins

30 g (1 oz) dry-roasted cashew nuts, coarsely chopped

CALORIES per muffin	150
60% Carbohydrate	24 g
13% Protein	5 g
27% Fat	5 g
CALCIUM	75 mg
IRON	2 mg
SODIUM	252 mg

Preheat the oven to 200°C (400°F or Mark 6). Lightly oil 12 deep bun tins or line them with paper liners. In a medium-sized bowl, stir together the oats, cereal and buttermilk; set aside for 30 minutes.

In another medium-sized bowl, cream together the margarine and sugar using an electric mixer. Beat in the egg, then stir in the flour, baking powder, bicarbonate of soda, salt and cinnamon. Add the flour mixture to the oat mixture and stir to combine. Stir in the courgettes, raisins and cashew nuts. Divide the batter among the tins and bake for 35 minutes, or until a toothpick inserted in the centre of a muffin comes out clean. Makes 12 muffins

Nutritionists recommend that your fluid intake should be about 2 litres (3½ pints), or six to eight glasses, per day. Some of this fluid should be in the form of plain water. But remember, too, that you get a fair amount of water from certain foods, especially vegetables, fruits and soups, as well as from other beverages.

CHEWY CITRUS THINS

Pack a few of these almost fat-free biscuits with a piece of fruit or a carton of fruit juice for an afternoon snack at work.

4 teaspoons margarine, melted and cooled

1 tablespoon lemon juice

2 teaspoons lime juice

45 g (1½ oz) plain flour

½ teaspoon grated lemon rind

¼ teaspoon grated lime rind

1 egg white

4 tablespoons sugar

Preheat the oven to 180°C (350°F or Mark 4). Line two baking sheets with lightly oiled foil and set aside. In a small bowl, stir together the margarine and lemon and lime juice; set aside. In another small bowl, combine the flour and lemon and lime rind. In a large bowl, beat the egg white until frothy using an electric mixer. Gradually add the sugar, continuing to beat on high speed for about 3 minutes, or until glossy peaks form; set aside. Sprinkle the flour mixture over the egg white and gently fold it in, then sprinkle the margarine mixture over the batter and fold it in. Using a level tablespoonful of batter for each one, form six biscuits on each baking sheet, spreading the batter into a 7.5 cm (3 inch) circle with the back of a spoon. Bake for 10 to 15 minutes, or until the biscuits are lightly browned round the edges. Let the biscuits cool on the baking sheet on a rack for 3 minutes, then peel them off the foil and place them on the rack to cool completely. Makes 12 biscuits

CALORIES per biscuit	40
65% Carbohydrate	7 g
10% Protein	1 g
25% Fat	1 g
CALCIUM	2 mg
IRON	Trace
SODIUM	19 mg

FRUIT-BOWL DRINK

If your schedule includes after-work exercise, this low-fat, high-carbohydrate beverage is an ideal snack before or after your session.

CALORIES per serving	70
95% Carbohydrate	18 g
5% Protein	1 g
0% Fat	0 g
CALCIUM	21 mg
IRON	1 mg
SODIUM	5 mg

30 cl (½ pint) orange juice
175 g (6 oz) seeded watermelon
   chunks
60 g (2 oz) fresh raspberries
75 g (2½ oz) fresh strawberries

75 g (2½ oz) fresh pineapple
   chunks
4 tablespoons unsweetened apple
   sauce
1 kiwi fruit, peeled
½ pear

Combine the ingredients in a food processor or blender and process until thick and smooth. Serve over ice in four tall glasses.   Makes 4 servings

SUNSET FRUIT MOULD

Packet jellies have about 4 teaspoons of sugar per serving. Making your own fruit jelly lets you control the sweetener, and a generous slice of this dessert gives you all the vitamin C you need daily.

125 g (4 oz) fresh raspberries or
   frozen unsweetened raspberries
1 grapefruit
1 orange
20 g (¾ oz) powdered gelatine

17.5 cl (6 fl oz) plain low-fat
   yogurt
3 tablespoons honey
30 cl (½ pint) apricot nectar
30 cl (½ pint) orange juice

CALORIES per serving	110
81% Carbohydrate	24 g
14% Protein	4 g
5% Fat	1 g
CALCIUM	61 mg
IRON	Trace
SODIUM	19 mg

Oil a 1.5 litre (2½ pint) ring mould; arrange eight raspberries in the bottom and set aside. Peel the grapefruit and orange, removing the white pith. Working over a bowl to catch the juice, segment the fruit; remove and discard the membranes. Cut the grapefruit segments in half; set aside the fruit and juice.

Place 17.5 cl (6 fl oz) of cold water in a small saucepan, sprinkle the gelatine over it and set aside for 5 minutes, then place over low heat and cook, stirring, for 5 minutes, or until the gelatine is dissolved. Combine the yogurt and 1½ tablespoons of honey in a small bowl and stir in 2 tablespoons of the gelatine mixture; set aside. In a large bowl, combine the remaining gelatine mixture, the apricot nectar, orange juice and remaining honey. Set the bowl in another large bowl half filled with iced water and allow it to stand, stirring occasionally, for 15 minutes, or until the mixture begins to thicken. Fold 17.5 cl (6 fl oz) of the fruit gelatine into the yogurt mixture and set aside.

Add the grapefruit and orange segments and their juice to the fruit gelatine and continue to chill it for about 20 minutes, or until it is thick enough to mound. Gently fold in the remaining raspberries and spoon the mixture into the prepared mould, levelling the surface with a spatula; refrigerate the mould. Place the bowl with the yogurt mixture in the bowl of iced water for 5 minutes, or until thickened, then spoon the yogurt mixture over the jelly in the mould, spreading it evenly. Refrigerate for 2 to 4 hours, or until firmly set.

To turn out the jelly, run a knife round the edge to loosen it. Invert the mould on a large plate and shake it gently. If the jelly does not fall out, place a towel wrung out in hot water over the inverted mould for about 1 minute, then gently shake the mould again.   Makes 8 servings

FRUIT FOLD-UPS

Resist the 300-calorie pastries on the office snack trolley, and treat yourself instead to one of these rich-tasting fruit-and-nut-filled biscuits.

150 g (5 oz) plain flour,
    approximately
2 tablespoons sugar
30 g (1 oz) margarine, well chilled
125 g (4 oz) low-fat cottage
    cheese

75 g (2½ oz) raisins
3 tablespoons coarsely chopped
    walnuts
¼ teaspoon ground cinnamon
¼ teaspoon pure vanilla extract
3 tablespoons strawberry jam

CALORIES per biscuit	85
65% Carbohydrate	14 g
10% Protein	2 g
25% Fat	3 g
CALCIUM	22 mg
IRON	Trace
SODIUM	47 mg

In a medium-sized bowl, stir together the flour and sugar. Using a pastry blender or two knives, cut in the margarine until the mixture resembles coarse crumbs. Stir in the cottage cheese, gather the dough into a ball and knead it a few times in the bowl, then cover it loosely and refrigerate for 1 hour. Combine the raisins and walnuts on a cutting board and chop them finely; transfer to a small bowl and stir in the cinnamon and vanilla extract.

Preheat the oven to 170°C (325°F or Mark 3). Line a large baking sheet with foil; set aside. Lightly flour the work surface and a rolling pin. Divide the dough in two; roll out each piece into a 12.5 by 30 cm (5 by 12 inch) rectangle and place one rectangle with a long side towards you. Brush the bottom half with half the jam, sprinkle it with half the raisin mixture and fold the top of the dough over to cover the filling. Cut the folded strip crosswise into eight equal biscuits. Place the biscuits 5 cm (2 inches) apart on the baking sheet and make eight more in the same way. Bake for 30 minutes, or until the biscuits are golden-brown, then transfer them to racks to cool.   Makes 16 biscuits

Fruit Fold-Ups

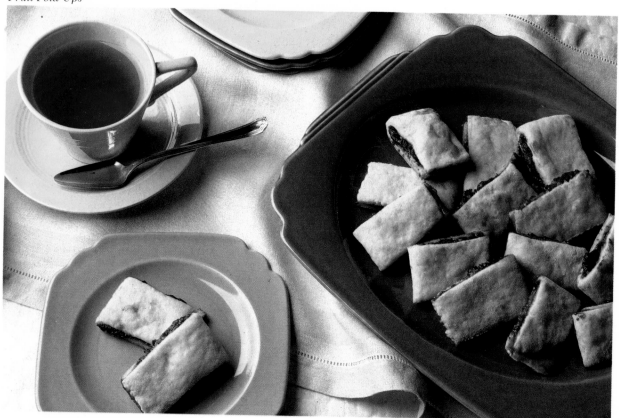

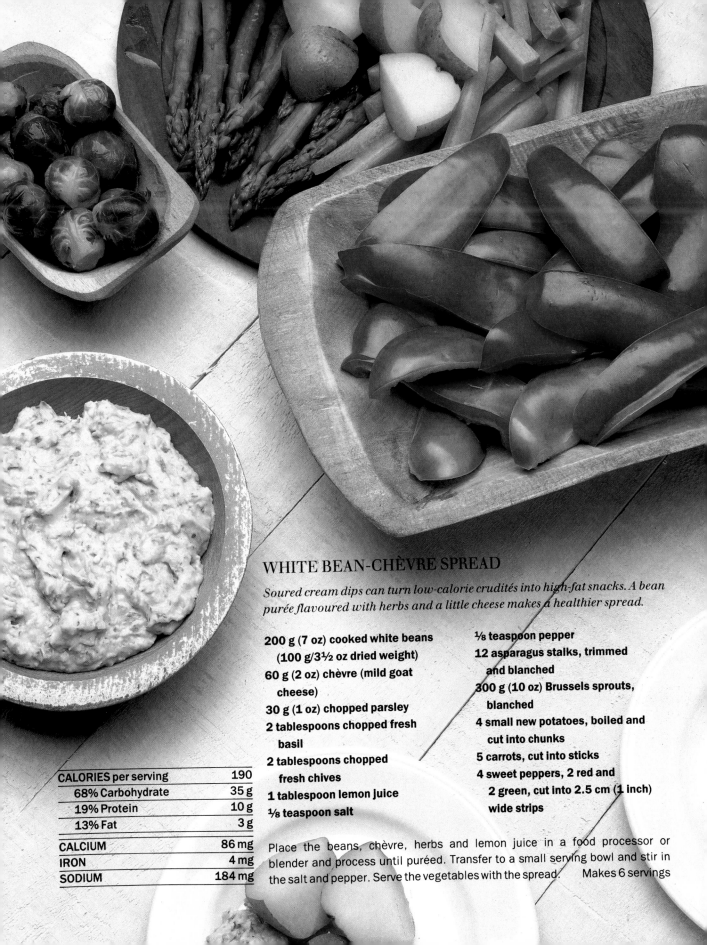

WHITE BEAN-CHÈVRE SPREAD

Soured cream dips can turn low-calorie crudités into high-fat snacks. A bean purée flavoured with herbs and a little cheese makes a healthier spread.

200 g (7 oz) cooked white beans
   (100 g/3½ oz dried weight)
60 g (2 oz) chèvre (mild goat
   cheese)
30 g (1 oz) chopped parsley
2 tablespoons chopped fresh
   basil
2 tablespoons chopped
   fresh chives
1 tablespoon lemon juice
⅛ teaspoon salt

⅛ teaspoon pepper
12 asparagus stalks, trimmed
   and blanched
300 g (10 oz) Brussels sprouts,
   blanched
4 small new potatoes, boiled and
   cut into chunks
5 carrots, cut into sticks
4 sweet peppers, 2 red and
   2 green, cut into 2.5 cm (1 inch)
   wide strips

Place the beans, chèvre, herbs and lemon juice in a food processor or blender and process until puréed. Transfer to a small serving bowl and stir in the salt and pepper. Serve the vegetables with the spread.   Makes 6 servings

CALORIES per serving	190
68% Carbohydrate	35 g
19% Protein	10 g
13% Fat	3 g
CALCIUM	86 mg
IRON	4 mg
SODIUM	184 mg

THREE-GRAIN BREADSTICKS

These peppery home-made breadsticks are satisfying between-meal snacks whether eaten alone or with a cup of soup or some low-fat cheese.

7 g (¼ oz) dried yeast
125 g (4 oz) wholemeal flour
150 g (5 oz) plain flour
60 g (2 oz) rye flour
½ teaspoon salt

1 teaspoon coarsely ground
  pepper
Pinch of cayenne pepper
2 tablespoons cornmeal

Place the yeast in a large bowl, add 25 cl (8 fl oz) of warm water (40-45°C/105-115°F) and cover the bowl with plastic film; set aside for 10 minutes. In another large bowl, combine the wholemeal, plain and rye flours, salt, pepper and cayenne pepper. Gradually stir the dry ingredients into the yeast mixture until a stiff dough forms. Turn the dough out on to a lightly floured work surface and knead it, adding a little more flour if necessary, for 8 to 10 minutes, or until the dough is smooth and elastic. Lightly oil the bowl, place the dough in the bowl, cover with a tea towel and leave to rise in a warm place for 1 to 1½ hours, or until the dough is doubled in bulk.

Preheat the oven to 180°C (350°F or Mark 4). Sprinkle two non-stick baking sheets lightly with cornmeal. Knock back the dough and knead it for 2 to 3 minutes, then let it rest for 10 minutes. Divide the dough into four, then divide each piece into 10 equal parts. With floured hands, roll each piece of dough into a stick about 30 cm (12 inches) long and 5 mm (¼ inch) thick. Place the breadsticks on the baking sheets and bake for 15 to 20 minutes, or until lightly browned, switching the position of the baking sheets half way through the baking time. Transfer the breadsticks to wire racks to cool, then leave at room temperature, uncovered, for 12 to 24 hours to crisp. Store the breadsticks loosely wrapped to keep them crisp.   Makes 40 breadsticks

CALORIES per breadstick	30
83% Carbohydrate	6 g
13% Protein	1 g
4% Fat	0.1 g
CALCIUM	3 mg
IRON	Trace
SODIUM	28 mg

DRIED FRUIT PATTIES

Prunes and other dried fruits are excellent sources of minerals and fibre, and their concentrated natural sweetness helps satisfy a sugar craving.

½ teaspoon vegetable oil
20 dried apricot halves
10 dried apple slices

10 whole stoned prunes
12 whole unblanched almonds

Lightly oil the bowl and blade of a food processor. Cut four apricot halves into 16 thin slices; set aside. Place the remaining apricot halves, the apple slices, prunes and almonds in the processor and process until very finely chopped: the mixture should form a cohesive mass. Moisten your hands and shape the fruit mixture into a 15 by 4 cm (6 by 1½ inch) log. Using a sharp knife dipped in hot water, cut the log into sixteen equal slices. If necessary, moisten your fingers again and reshape the slices into round patties. Place the patties on a baking sheet and press an apricot strip into the top of each one. Cover with plastic film and store the patties in the refrigerator.   Makes 16 patties

Note: if you do not have a food processor, the ingredients can be chopped by hand. Lightly oil the knife blade to help keep the fruit from sticking to it.

CALORIES per patty	45
73% Carbohydrate	9 g
6% Protein	1 g
21% Fat	1 g
CALCIUM	10 mg
IRON	Trace
SODIUM	4 mg

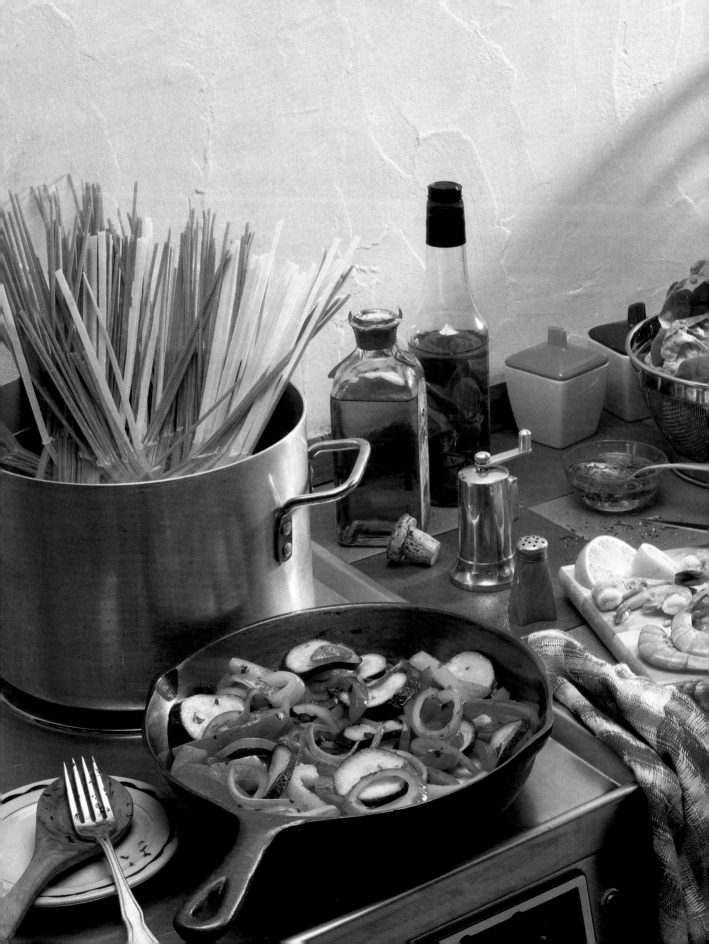

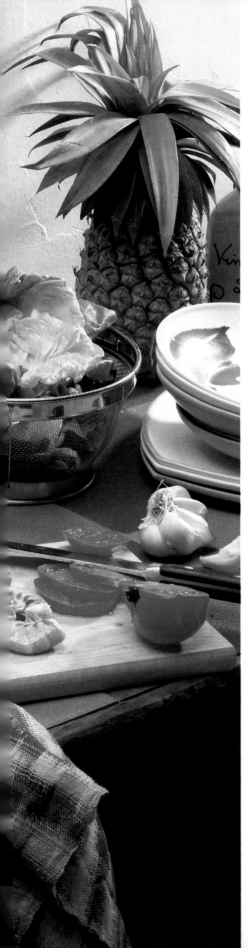

CHAPTER FOUR

Dinner

*Behaviour-modification
strategies, alternatives to meat,
low-calorie desserts*

Limiting calorie intake at dinner is one of the most important elements of a successful weight-loss and maintenance programme. This meal, which can include an appetizer, main course, one or two side dishes, bread or rolls, beverage and dessert, usually constitutes the largest of the day. Although those on a weight-control plan sometimes skip breakfast or lunch, only rarely do they omit dinner. Most nutritionists recommend, however, that calorie consumption be more evenly distributed throughout the day.

The evening meal can be a difficult time for people who are cutting calories not only because of the amount of food offered to them, but also because of dinner's social aspect. An American survey found that almost 80 per cent of American dinners are eaten with household members. And because this meal occurs at a time of day when you can

put work-related pressures aside and relax, dinner tends to be a more leisurely meal than either breakfast or lunch — which may greatly increase the temptation to overeat.

You can take steps to resist that temptation. In fact, the social aspect of dinner can actually aid you in eating smaller amounts. Put down your utensils between bites and make a point of talking to your companions. This will help you to avoid excessively fast eating, a factor that has been linked with obesity. Another effective behaviour-modification strategy is to condition yourself always to leave some food uneaten, which may be difficult at first if you were raised with the directive to finish everything on your plate.

You can also alter your eating environment when you eat at home. Remove the temptation for second helpings by having one person serve food from the kitchen, rather than serving at the table. And switch from standard to smaller-sized dinner plates to give the illusion of more food on each plate.

In order to satisfy your appetite with low-calorie food, begin your dinner with a low-fat soup or a crunchy, fresh vegetable salad. Several recent studies have found that soup eaten before a meal will fill your stomach and so lead to lower total calorie consumption for the meal. Both this chapter and the preceding one include several recipes for soups that are low in calories but rich in nutrients. Likewise, the fibre contained in raw vegetables such as sweet red peppers and carrots — used in the Two-Rice and Pasta Salad on page 140 — will start to fill you up before you get to the main course.

Although the consumption of poultry has escalated in the United Kingdom in the past two decades, many dinners still centre round servings of high-fat red meat that total 250 grams or more. Apart from the nutritional harm that the saturated fat in meat causes, particularly with regard to raising your cholesterol level, most red meat is very high in calories. A 250 gram T-bone steak, for example, derives 60 per cent of its 555 calories from fat. A 250 gram chicken breast with the skin intact contributes 450 calories, of which nearly 40 per cent are fat. Removing all visible fat from meat and the skin from poultry will significantly reduce their calorie and fat content. Far more effective than trimming fat from meat and poultry is to eat more low-fat fish and seafood, such as the Marinated Scallop Kebabs on page 118, instead. You can also substitute high-fibre grains for your main dishes.

Many of the recipes that follow show you how to use meat as an adjunct to a meal, rather than as the centrepiece, with appetizing results that are low in calories. The Pilaff with Marinated Steak on page 134, for example, uses only 37 grams of meat per portion, enough to give the dish a hearty flavour and some iron and B vitamins.

Besides containing a considerable portion of meat, many conventional dinner dishes are cooked in butter or oil, while others feature heavy cream sauces, marinades and stuffings — all of which add unneeded fat. Cooking in a non-stick frying pan and substituting wine,

▼ Most of the main-dish recipes in this chapter have from 300 to 395 calories per serving. Certain recipes, marked with a triangle, are extra-low in calories — between 170 and 275 per serving. Such recipes can be eaten as main dishes or combined with other foods. Three side dishes, all of which contain fewer than 150 calories, are also included. The desserts in this chapter all have fewer than 275 calories.

Desserts

A considerable percentage of excess calories in the diet comes from fat and sugar-laden desserts. In fact, most Britons get about one fifth of their total daily calories from sugar. Giving up desserts is not necessary for a successful diet, but modifying your dessert choices may be. The following tips will help you lower your dessert calories:

◆ Choose fruit, either fresh or in combinations such as compotes, in place of cakes, biscuits and other baked goods, most of which are high in fat and heavily sweetened. You can make a fruit-yogurt parfait by alternating layers of the two ingredients. If you have canned fruit, check the label to see that it is canned in its own juice or in water, not sweetened syrup. To add variety to fruit desserts, stew or purée the fruit with cinnamon, nutmeg or other spices. Another possibility is to freeze fruits such as grapes or bananas; eat them straight from the freezer, rather than thawing them which makes their texture mushy.

◆ Decrease the sugar you use when you bake at home. In most recipes, sugar can be reduced by a third to a half without compromising the flavour of the dessert. Substituting brown sugar for white sugar does not reduce calories — they are equal in calorie content, 16 calories per teaspoon, and equally devoid of vitamins and minerals. When you buy commercially prepared baked goods, make a habit of reading the labels. Fructose, dextrose, maltose, sucrose, corn syrup, sorbitol, xylitol and mannitol are all forms of sugar.

◆ Instead of a bowl of ice cream, finish your meal with a fruit-based sorbet. Sorbet contains approximately half the calories of dairy ice cream and less than 1 per cent fat. Another option is low-fat frozen yogurt, with approximately 25 per cent fewer calories than ice cream. Better still are frozen fruit bars: those made with just fruit and fruit juice average only 70 calories per serving.

◆ If you have always thought of dessert as a reward for yourself, try to modify your behaviour to focus on other non-food pleasures. Get into the habit of taking a walk after dinner with family and friends, for example, or reading a magazine or a book.

bouillon, lemon juice or soy sauce for oil or butter are important steps for preparing low-calorie dinner dishes. The trout recipe given on page 130, for example, features a vegetable stuffing that does not depend on butter for flavour. Using lemon juice, yogurt and spices as salad dressings or as toppings for baked potatoes will also help you keep the number of calories you consume in check.

In addition to dessert recipes that are low in calories offered throughout this chapter, substitutions are suggested in the box above to enable you to include other desserts without paying the traditional toll in excess fat and sugar. Finally, one of the most difficult situations you may face while trying to lose weight is deciding what to eat when you are in a restaurant; the following two pages will guide you through menu choices and provide suggestions for eating at parties and other social occasions.

Dining Out

Many, if not most, people who embark on a weight-loss programme find that dining out in restaurants can become their biggest challenge. As the chart on the opposite page indicates, a fair number of traditional menu main courses and side dishes are high in fat. And restaurants often increase the fat content of a dish by the way they prepare it — drenching a salad in an oily dressing, for example, or adding a mound of whipped cream to a piece of pie.

At the same time, there is a growing awareness among restaurant owners and food franchisers that the public is interested in low-fat, low-calorie alternatives to traditional menu selections. In a recent study conducted by an American public-opinion organization, more than half of the 500 restaurant managers surveyed reported an increased demand for salads and seafood dishes. Three quarters of the respondents also maintained that they would alter their food-preparation methods if their customers asked them to do so.

The keys to dining out without overeating — be it at a restaurant, a party or a business gathering — are planning ahead and not allowing your motivation to falter. Here are some suggestions on how you can retain habits to help you control your weight when not eating at home:

• Before you go out for a meal, have a low-calorie snack. Raw vegetables, a piece of fruit or a slice of low-fat cheese will help fill you up so that you are not tempted by the richer foods you may be offered at a restaurant or party.

• Resist alcoholic drinks before, during and after dinner, or limit yourself to a glass of wine or beer. Exercising moderation has merit not only as a way in which to avoid unneeded calories: more than one drink tends to undermine your determination to restrain your eating. Of course, you can drink as much water before and during your meal as you want.

• Eat a few slices of bread before your dinner, preferably wholemeal bread, spread with a minimum of butter or margarine. Bread itself is low in fat and is relatively low in calories for its volume.

• Ask to have salad dressings served separately. Avoid such toppings as olives, avocado and bacon, which are high in fat. If possible, make your own salad dressing of vinegar, oil, and spices. Some of the most popular dressings that are served in restaurants are mayonnaise or soured cream-based, and they get 90 per cent of their calories from fat.

• Try to choose entrées and accompaniments chiefly from the centre column on the opposite page. Use your judgment — and the recipes in this book — to identify other dishes that are comparatively low in fat.

• Ask your waiter how certain foods are prepared. If the menu lists fried fish fillets, for example, you can ask that your fish be grilled with lemon juice instead of butter. You may be able to have such dishes as lobster Newburg served with a minimum amount of sauce, or with the sauce served separately. Some restaurants will cook chicken with the skin removed on request.

• Order fresh fruit for dessert. Fruit has more vitamins, minerals and fibre than ice cream, cake or pie, and most fruits contain no fat.

WHAT TO ORDER

Choosing wisely from a menu is more than a matter of self-denial for those who are weight-conscious. If you prefer foods that get less than 30 per cent of their calories from fat, select your meal from the middle column; the left-hand column contains items that are from 30 to 60 per cent fat. The foods in the right-hand column are more than 60 per cent fat.

OCCASIONALLY

Poached salmon, with low-fat sauce

Chicken, dark meat, no skin

Turkey, dark meat, no skin

Duck, no skin

Devilled crab

Lobster Newburg

Grilled rump steak

Lean pork tenderloin

Mashed potatoes

OFTEN

White fish, steamed, poached or grilled without fat

Chicken, white meat, no skin

Lean roast topside

Roast venison

Grilled prawns

Steamed lobster

Spaghetti with tomato sauce

Baked potato with any low-fat topping

Steamed vegetables

Green salad with low-fat yogurt dressing

RARELY

Fried chicken (including nuggets)

Deep-fried prawns

Corned beef and processed meats

Roast leg of lamb

Braised steak with gravy

Pork spareribs

Coleslaw

Fried onion rings

Chips

Aerobic Workouts

Many studies have confirmed that aerobic exercise is the most efficient form of activity to burn off calories and thereby lose unwanted fat. For an exercise to be aerobic, it must provide continuous exertion for your body's major muscle groups. In order to cause the loss of body fat, the exercise must be performed for a long enough time to expend a significant number of calories. All endurance activities, such as running, cross-country skiing, cycling, swimming and rowing, are aerobic exercises. Certain racket sports can also produce a high calorie output if they are played intensely enough and at a sustained rhythm. The chart opposite indicates the calorie values for different aerobic activities.

Based on guidelines established by the American College of Sports Medicine, you should exercise at least four days a week for 40 to 50 minutes, at a pace that raises your heart rate to within 60 to 75 per cent of its maximum. If you are in good shape, you may do shorter, less frequent workouts at a slightly higher intensity: three days per week for 20 to 30 minutes per session, maintaining an intensity of at least 80 to 85 per cent of your maximum heart rate. (These recommended times do not include warm-up and cool-down.) Studies have shown that such a schedule is the minimum for any noticeable change in body weight or composition to occur.

To determine if you are exercising at the proper intensity, count your pulse for 10 seconds and multiply by six to obtain your heart rate. While you exercise, your heart rate should fall within a target zone that is 60 to 85 per cent of its estimated maximum — which you can calculate by subtracting your age from 220. If you are 35 years old, for example, your target heart rate zone falls between 111 and 157 beats per minute.

During your workout, check your heart rate periodically to make sure you are exercising within your target heart rate zone. Once you have become accustomed to this level of intensity, you will begin to recognize when you have reached it without checking your pulse.

At each workout, you should warm up by performing your activity at an easy pace for five minutes, then build up the intensity. Exercise for at least 20 minutes within your target heart rate zone. Spend five minutes cooling down by gradually reducing the intensity of your workout.

The hardest part of an exercise programme is doing it regularly. If running bores you, the chances are that forcing yourself to complete a daily 8-kilometre run will ultimately lead you to give it up. Instead, choose an exercise that you enjoy and that is accessible to you. The chart on the opposite page lists some of the benefits that various exercises provide. You can also consider cross-training, or alternating two or more activities, such as cycling and cross-country skiing.

An Exercise Guide

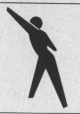

AEROBIC DANCE

This activity works all of your major muscles and can be performed either at home or in classes. If done at home, you can set your pace by your choice of music: fast-tempo music will make the session more vigorous. Ensure that your workouts are low-impact — one foot should be on the floor at all times — to reduce your chances of injury.

Light:	120
Moderate:	200
Vigorous:	300

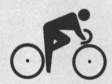

CYCLING

A superb conditioner for the lower body, cycling can be performed outdoors or on an indoor stationary bike that allows you to adjust how hard you pedal. Outdoors, the injury rate is low, though cyclists should always wear hard-shell helmets for safety.

9 km/h:	130
16 km/h:	220
21 km/h:	320

RACKET SPORTS

Unlike the rhythmic movements of other aerobic activities, racket sports alternate high and low-intensity movements. Squash, racketball and singles tennis are most effective for burning calories and for overall conditioning.

Badminton:	175
Tennis:	210
Racketball:	360
Squash:	420

RUNNING

A highly efficient exercise, running is also convenient and inexpensive. Competitive long-distance runners have less body fat than any other group of athletes. Running places stress on the knees, lower legs and feet, so be sure to wear good running shoes that fit correctly.

9 km/h:	320
10 km/h:	350
12 km/h:	430
16 km/h:	550

SKIING

Both downhill and cross-country skiing can be excellent conditioners. Cross-country burns calories more efficiently since you need not stop at the bottom of each hill. Cross-country skiing also strengthens the shoulders and upper arms.

Downhill:	300
Cross-country:	200-560

SWIMMING

Many people, especially those who are overweight, find swimming an enjoyable exercise because it is free of weight-bearing stresses. The front crawl, or "freestyle" is the most efficient stroke for an aerobic workout as well as being a good upper body conditioner.

25 m/min:	165
40 m/min:	240
50 m/min:	345

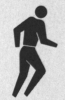

WALKING

Certainly the most accessible exercise activity, walking is ideal if you are just starting an exercise programme. You can increase the caloric expenditure of walking by increasing your pace and vigorously swinging your arms. Fast walking can burn more calories than running.

4 km/h:	105
7 km/h:	200
10 km/h:	370

*Approximate caloric expenditure for a person weighing 68 kilograms. Add 10 per cent for every 7 kilograms over this weight and subtract 10 per cent for every 7 kilograms under.

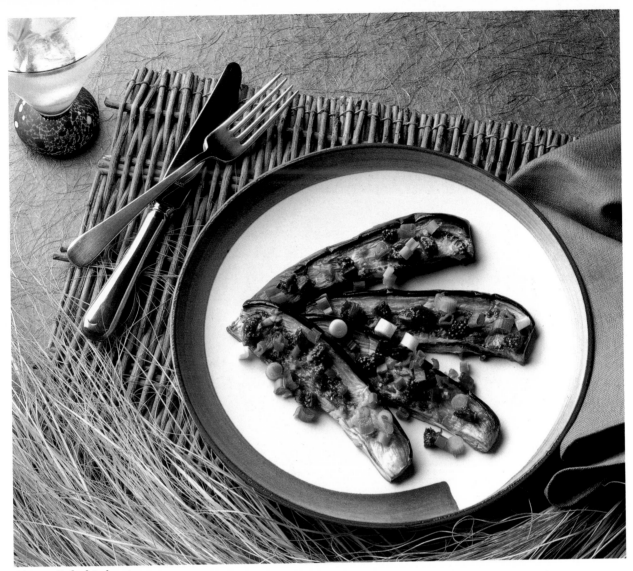

Chinese Baked Aubergine

CHINESE BAKED AUBERGINE ▼

A little chicken stock (instead of a lot of oil) keeps the aubergine moist during cooking. The sesame oil in this recipe is mainly for flavour.

750 g (1½ lb) aubergine
1 tablespoon sesame oil
1 tablespoon finely chopped fresh
   ginger root
2 garlic cloves, chopped
Pinch of salt

Pepper
12.5 cl (4 fl oz) low-sodium
   chicken stock
60 g (2 oz) dried figs, chopped
60 g (2 oz) spring onions,
   chopped

CALORIES per serving	235
65% Carbohydrate	42 g
9% Protein	6 g
26% Fat	8 g
CALCIUM	186 mg
IRON	3 mg
SODIUM	96 mg

Preheat the oven to 190°C (375°F or Mark 5). Line a baking sheet with foil. Trim the aubergine and cut it in half lengthwise. Cut the halves lengthwise into 1 cm (½ inch) thick slices, lay them on the baking sheet and sprinkle with the oil, ginger, garlic, salt and pepper to taste. Dribble the chicken stock over the aubergine, scatter the figs on top and bake for 30 minutes, or until the figs are golden-brown. Top with the spring onions and serve.   Makes 2 servings

HERBED FETTUCCINE

If you find that a small portion of chicken or fish and a salad is not a filling meal, add a side dish of complex carbohydrates such as this lightly sauced pasta.

3 garlic cloves
60 g (2 oz) fresh basil leaves
2 tablespoons olive oil

12.5 cl (4 fl oz) low-sodium
  chicken stock
250 g (8 oz) dried fettuccine

CALORIES per serving	150
60% Carbohydrate	22 g
11% Protein	4 g
29% Fat	5 g
CALCIUM	59 mg
IRON	2 mg
SODIUM	6 mg

Preheat the oven to 200°C (400°F or Mark 6). Place the unpeeled garlic cloves on a sheet of foil and bake them for 10 to 15 minutes, or until golden-brown. Let the garlic cool slightly, then remove and discard the peel. Place the garlic cloves and basil in a food processor or blender and process for 15 to 30 seconds, or until finely chopped. With the machine running, slowly add the oil and stock; set aside.

Bring a large pan of water to the boil. Add the fettuccine and cook it for 10 to 12 minutes, or according to the packet directions until *al dente*. Drain the pasta and transfer it to a serving bowl; toss with the sauce. Serve immediately or, to serve chilled, refrigerate for at least 3 hours.   Makes 8 servings

MOROCCAN STEW

Ethnic dishes add interest to a diet. Chick-peas are a good source of folic acid, a vitamin necessary for red blood cell production.

250 g (8 oz) acorn squash
1 courgette
1 onion
2 carrots
25 cl (8 fl oz) low-sodium
  chicken stock
125 g (4 oz) skinless boneless
  chicken breast
400 g (14 oz) canned plum
  tomatoes, with their liquid

90 g (3 oz) cooked chick-peas
4 tablespoons raisins or currants
2 teaspoons vegetable oil
¼ teaspoon salt
⅛ teaspoon ground cinnamon
Dash of Tabasco sauce
250 g (8 oz) couscous
2 tablespoons toasted flaked
  almonds
1 tablespoon chopped fresh mint

CALORIES per serving	390
66% Carbohydrate	59 g
21% Protein	19 g
13% Fat	5 g
CALCIUM	102 mg
IRON	3 mg
SODIUM	350 mg

Peel and seed the acorn squash and cut it into 1 cm (½ inch) dice. Trim the courgette and peel the onion and cut them into 5 mm (¼ inch) dice. Peel and trim the carrots and cut them into 5 mm (¼ inch) thick diagonal slices.

Put the acorn squash, onion, carrots and stock in a medium-sized sauce-pan, cover and cook over medium heat for 10 minutes, or until the vegetables are tender but still crisp. Meanwhile, cut the chicken into 2.5 cm (1 inch) dice. Add the chicken, the courgette, the tomatoes and their liquid, the chick-peas, raisins, oil, salt, cinnamon and Tabasco sauce and cook, uncovered, over me-dium heat for 5 minutes, or until the vegetables are tender and the chicken is cooked. Meanwhile, bring 50 cl (16 fl oz) of water to the boil in a medium-sized saucepan. Stir in the couscous with a wire whisk and cook for 30 sec-onds. Remove from the heat; cover the pan and let it stand for 7 minutes.

To serve, fluff the couscous with a fork and mound it on a serving platter. Spoon the chicken mixture over the couscous and sprinkle it with the almonds and mint.   Makes 4 servings

CALORIES per serving	195
52% Carbohydrate	26 g
28% Protein	14 g
20% Fat	5 g
CALCIUM	57 mg
IRON	3 mg
SODIUM	261 mg

MARINATED SCALLOP KEBABS ▼

This Mexican-style dish is a variation on seviche, which is made with uncooked seafood. This low-calorie meal supplies about one quarter of your protein requirement and all the vitamins A and C you need daily.

250 g (8 oz) scallops, cleaned
125 g (4 oz) cherry tomatoes
12.5 cl (4 fl oz) freshly squeezed
  orange juice
3 tablespoons freshly
  squeezed lemon juice
1 tablespoon olive oil
1 tablespoon grated orange rind

2 tablespoons chopped
  fresh coriander
1 large sweet yellow or red
  pepper
250 g (8 oz) broccoli florets,
  blanched
Four 30 g (1 oz) rye bread rolls

Bring 50 cl (16 fl oz) of water to the boil in a small saucepan. Add the scallops, reduce the heat to low and simmer for 1 to 2 minutes, or until they are opaque and just firm; drain the scallops and place them in a medium-sized non-reactive bowl. Add the tomatoes, orange juice, lemon juice, oil, orange rind and coriander, and stir to combine. Stem and seed the sweet pepper, cut it into 2.5 cm (1 inch) squares and add it to the marinade. Add the broccoli, cover the bowl and place it in the refrigerator to marinate for 2 hours.

To serve, thread the scallops, tomatoes, broccoli and pepper alternately on eight long skewers and serve with the rolls.   Makes 4 servings

BEAN SOUP PAPRIKASH

CALORIES per serving	320
67% Carbohydrate	57 g
22% Protein	18 g
11% Fat	4 g
CALCIUM	157 mg
IRON	6 mg
SODIUM	181 mg

If you overeat because you rush through your meals, have soup more often. A study has shown that soup is eaten more slowly than other foods, thereby giving the brain more time to acknowledge that the stomach is full.

175 g (6 oz) dried kidney beans	1 teaspoon dry mustard
125 g (4 oz) dried pinto beans	1 litre (1¾ pints) low-sodium
2 large onions, peeled	beef stock
2 large garlic cloves, peeled	450 g (15 oz) canned chopped
500 g (1 lb) potatoes	tomatoes, with their liquid
2 large carrots	2½ tablespoons barley
175 g (6 oz) cabbage	4 tablespoons red wine vinegar
1 rasher smoked bacon, diced	Pepper to taste
2 tablespoons paprika	4 tablespoons thick Greek yogurt

Put the beans in a medium-sized saucepan, add 75 cl (1¼ pints) of water and bring to a simmer over medium heat. Cook for 2 minutes, then remove from the heat, cover and let stand for 1 hour. Drain the beans, add one onion, one garlic clove and 50 cl (16 fl oz) of water; bring to the boil and boil for 10 minutes. Reduce the heat to low and simmer for 1 hour, or until the beans are almost tender. Meanwhile, chop the remaining onion and garlic. Scrub the potatoes and cut them into 2.5 cm (1 inch) cubes. Trim, peel and slice the carrots. Trim the cabbage and cut it into 2.5 cm (1 inch) chunks; set aside.

Sauté the bacon in a large stockpot until browned. Add the chopped onion and garlic and cook for 5 minutes, or until soft. Add the stock, tomatoes, paprika and mustard and bring the soup to the boil. Add the barley, potatoes and carrots and cook for 45 minutes.

Add the beans and their liquid to the soup; remove and discard the whole onion and garlic. Add the cabbage and cook for about 15 minutes. Stir in the vinegar and pepper. Garnish with the yogurt and serve.　　Makes 6 servings

F*or cooking, use unhydrogenated oils that are high in polyunsaturated or monounsaturated fats. Safflower, sunflower, corn, soya bean, cottonseed and olive oils are good choices. But bear in mind that despite the nutritional advantage of non-saturated fats, all oils are 100 per cent fat and have the same calorie count — about 120 calories per tablespoon.*

BROWN RICE SAUTÉ ▼

The vegetables in a serving of this dish provide half your daily vitamin A, and, with the walnuts and brown rice, a good deal of fibre.

1 tablespoon corn oil	100 g (3½ oz) spring onions,
1 garlic clove, chopped	chopped
375 g (13 oz) cooked brown rice	Pinch of salt
(150 g/5 oz raw)	¼ teaspoon pepper
125 g (4 oz) courgettes, sliced	15 g (½ oz) walnut halves
150 g (5 oz) sweet red pepper,	1 tablespoon grated orange rind
diced	1 tablespoon chopped parsley

CALORIES per serving	220
65% Carbohydrate	36 g
8% Protein	5 g
27% Fat	7 g
CALCIUM	44 mg
IRON	2 mg
SODIUM	36 mg

Heat the oil in a medium-sized frying pan over medium heat. Add the garlic, and sauté for 2 to 3 minutes. Add the rice, courgettes, red pepper, spring onions, salt, pepper and 4 tablespoons of water and bring the mixture to the boil over high heat. Reduce the heat to medium low and simmer, stirring constantly, for 5 minutes, or until the courgettes and peppers are tender. Stir in the walnuts, orange rind and parsley and serve.　　Makes 4 servings

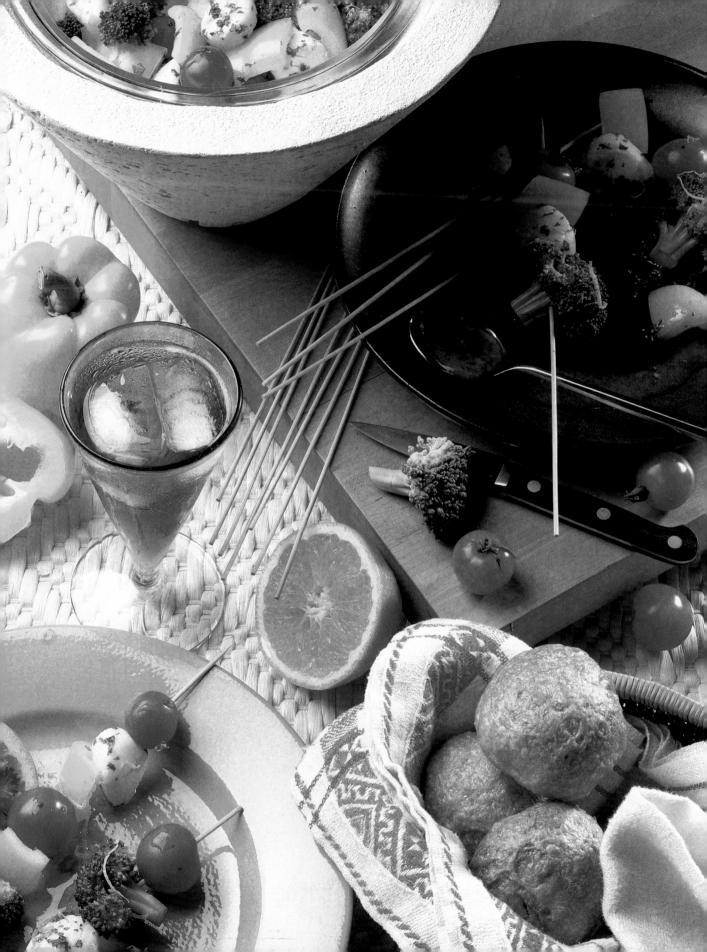

GREEK SALAD ▼

Eliminating the oil and olives from a Greek salad cuts fat and calories considerably; a yogurt dressing and black-eyed peas are used instead.

1 large cucumber
12.5 cl (4 fl oz) plain low-fat yogurt
4 tablespoons chopped fresh mint
3 tablespoons lemon juice
1 teaspoon sugar
4 plum tomatoes

125 g (4 oz) cos lettuce, torn into bite-sized pieces
325 g (11 oz) cooked black-eyed peas (150 g/5 oz dried weight)
30 g (1 oz) spring onions, chopped
30 g (1 oz) feta cheese, crumbled

CALORIES per serving	170
63% Carbohydrate	28 g
24% Protein	11 g
13% Fat	3 g
CALCIUM	142 mg
IRON	3 mg
SODIUM	123 mg

For the dressing, scrub the cucumber and halve it lengthwise. Peel and seed one half, cut it into large chunks and process it in a food processor or blender for 15 to 20 seconds, or until puréed. Add the yogurt, mint, lemon juice and sugar and process for another 5 to 10 seconds, scraping down the sides of the container with a rubber spatula; set aside. Cut the remaining cucumber half lengthwise into quarters, then cut it crosswise into 5 mm (¼ inch) thick slices. Cut the tomatoes into large dice. Place the lettuce, cucumber, tomatoes, black-eyed peas and spring onions in a large bowl and toss to combine. Sprinkle the feta cheese over the salad and, just before serving, add the dressing and toss the salad.   Makes 4 servings

Greek Salad

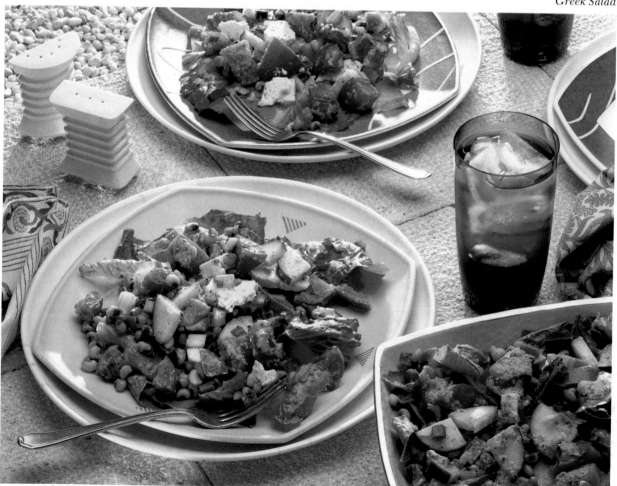

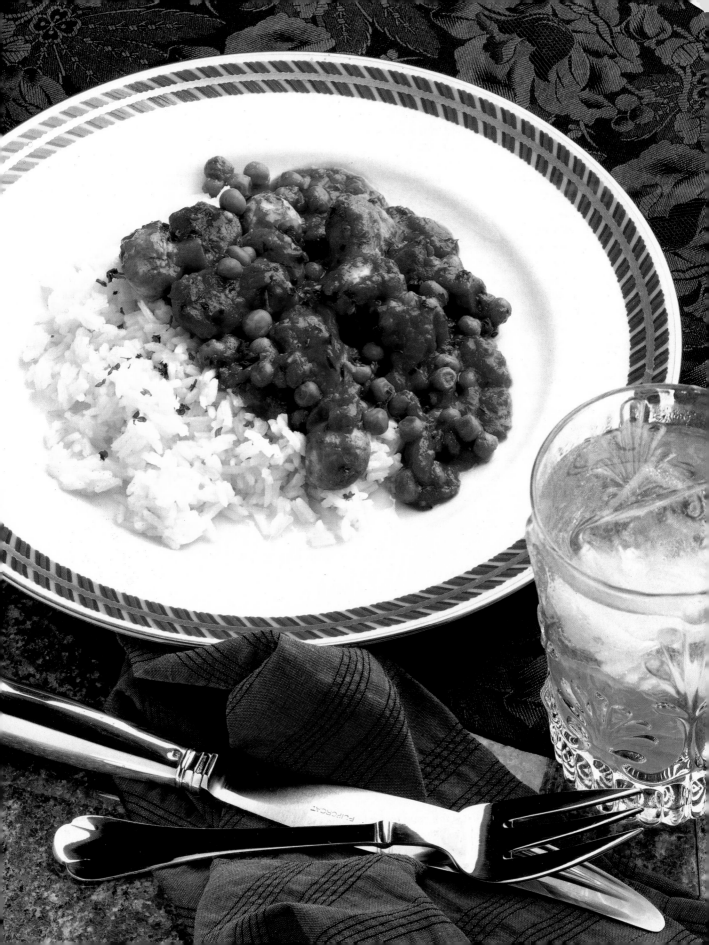

LAMB AND MUSHROOM STEW WITH ROSEMARY

*Low-fat diets often lack niacin, which helps the body use energy from foods.
This stew supplies more than half of a woman's daily niacin quota.*

2 tablespoons plain flour
¼ teaspoon salt
¼ teaspoon pepper
250 g (8 oz) lean stewing lamb,
   cut into 2.5 cm (1 inch) cubes
1 tablespoon vegetable oil
400 g (14 oz) canned plum
   tomatoes, with their liquid
125 g (4 oz) small mushrooms

1 garlic clove, crushed
1 bay leaf
¾ teaspoon fresh rosemary, or
   ¼ teaspoon dried rosemary,
   chopped
2 tablespoons chopped parsley
175 g (6 oz) long-grain white rice
75 g (2½ oz) frozen peas,
   thawed

CALORIES per serving	350
59% Carbohydrate	51 g
19% Protein	17 g
22% Fat	8 g
CALCIUM	61 mg
IRON	4 mg
SODIUM	339 mg

Mix the flour, salt and pepper on a sheet of greaseproof paper and dredge the lamb cubes in the mixture. Reserve the excess flour. Heat the oil in a medium-sized saucepan over medium heat, add the lamb and sauté for 5 to 10 minutes, or until the meat is well browned all over.

Add the remaining flour mixture and cook, stirring, for 1 minute. Add the tomatoes and their liquid, the mushrooms, garlic, bay leaf, rosemary and half the parsley and bring to the boil. Reduce the heat to medium low, cover the pan and simmer for 30 minutes. Meanwhile, bring 75 cl (1¼ pints) of water to the boil in a medium-sized saucepan. Stir in the rice, cover the pan, reduce the heat to medium low and simmer for 20 minutes, or until the rice is tender and the water is completely absorbed. Remove the bay leaf from the stew and stir in the peas. Divide the rice among four plates, spoon the stew over it and sprinkle with the remaining parsley.   *Makes 4 servings*

CAULIFLOWER-CHEESE SOUP

A bowl of this thick puréed soup supplies your full daily requirement of vitamin C, most of it from the sweet potato and cauliflower.

1 tablespoon butter
100 g (3½ oz) leeks, chopped
50 cl (16 fl oz) low-sodium
   chicken stock
400 g (14 oz) orange-fleshed
   sweet potato, peeled and cut into
   1 cm (½ inch) thick slices

400 g (14 oz) cauliflower florets
1 tablespoon grainy mustard
2 tablespoons chopped parsley
45 g (1½ oz) Emmenthal cheese,
   grated
4 small pitta breads

If you love cheese, it is hard to give it up for a low-fat diet; however, if you select cheese carefully and limit the amount you eat, you can still cut fat and calories. Almost all hard cheeses are high in fat, but if you choose sharp, strong-flavoured mature ones such as Cheddar or Parmesan, just a sprinkling is enough.

Heat the butter in a medium-sized saucepan over medium heat. Add the leeks, and sauté for 3 to 5 minutes, or until tender. Add the stock and 25 cl (8 fl oz) of water and bring to the boil. Add the sweet potato and cauliflower, reduce the heat to low, cover the pan and simmer for about 20 minutes, or until the sweet potato is tender.

Remove the pan from the heat and allow the soup to cool slightly. Process the soup in a food processor or blender for 1 to 2 minutes, or until puréed, scraping down the sides of the container with a rubber spatula. Stir in the mustard and parsley, ladle the soup into four bowls and top each one with the cheese. Serve with the pitta breads, warmed if desired.   *Makes 4 servings*

CALORIES per serving	320
67% Carbohydrate	54 g
15% Protein	12 g
18% Fat	7 g
CALCIUM	166 mg
IRON	3 mg
SODIUM	418 mg

◁ *Lamb and Mushroom Stew with Rosemary*

ITALIAN SPLIT-PEA STEW

Without the traditional ham or sausage, split-pea stew becomes a low-fat dish; it is also an excellent source of B vitamins, potassium and fibre.

CALORIES per serving	340
67% Carbohydrate	61 g
20% Protein	18 g
13% Fat	5 g
CALCIUM	133 mg
IRON	5 mg
SODIUM	604 mg

15 g (½ oz) butter
250 g (8 oz) onions, chopped
1 garlic clove, chopped
1.1 kg (36 oz) canned plum tomatoes, with their liquid

200 g (7 oz) dried yellow split peas
¾ teaspoon dried oregano
1 bay leaf
4 wholemeal rolls (60 g/2 oz each)

Heat the butter in a medium-sized saucepan over medium heat. Add the onions and garlic and sauté for 10 minutes, or until golden. Add the tomatoes and their liquid, the split peas, oregano, bay leaf and 25 cl (8 fl oz) of water and bring to the boil. Reduce the heat to medium low, cover the pan and simmer the stew for 25 minutes, or until the peas are tender. Ten minutes before serving, warm the rolls in a 180°C (350°F or Mark 4) oven.

To serve, remove and discard the bay leaf, ladle the stew into four bowls and eat with the warm rolls. Makes 4 servings

LENTILS WITH GOAT CHEESE DRESSING

Combining lentils, which are pulses, with a grain such as brown rice gives you complete protein: the amino acids lacking in the lentils are supplied by the rice. Adding cheese and chicken stock, which are complete proteins, further enhances your protein intake from this meal.

CALORIES per serving	295
53% Carbohydrate	40 g
17% Protein	13 g
30% Fat	10 g
CALCIUM	121 mg
IRON	5 mg
SODIUM	386 mg

200 g (7 oz) dried lentils
350 g (12 oz) red onions, diced
60 g (2 oz) spring onions, finely chopped
125 g (4 oz) carrots, grated
150 g (5 oz) cooked brown rice (60 g/2 oz raw)
1 teaspoon grated lemon rind
12.5 cl (4 fl oz) low-sodium chicken stock
4 tablespoons red wine vinegar, preferably balsamic

3 tablespoons vegetable oil
2 teaspoons Dijon mustard
60 g (2 oz) mild goat cheese
½ teaspoon salt
Pepper to taste
250 g (8 oz) red cabbage, thinly sliced
250 g (8 oz) spinach, shredded
100 g (3½ oz) sweet red pepper, slivered
90 g (3 oz) radishes, julienned
30 g (1 oz) parsley, finely chopped

Place the lentils and 75 cl (1¼ pints) of water in a medium-sized saucepan and bring to the boil over medium heat. Reduce the heat to low and simmer for about 25 minutes, or until the lentils are soft. Drain any liquid and transfer the lentils to a medium-sized bowl to cool. Add the red onions, spring onions, carrots, rice and lemon rind and toss to combine; set aside.

For the dressing, process the stock, vinegar, oil, mustard, cheese, salt and pepper in a food processor until well blended. Pour it over the lentil mixture and stir to combine; set aside for 30 minutes to allow the flavours to blend.

To serve, make a bed of cabbage and spinach on a large serving platter and mound the lentil salad on top. Garnish with the red pepper, radishes and parsley and serve. Makes 6 servings

124

CABBAGE-CARROT-BEAN SOUP

A serving of this soup has only 188 milligrams of sodium, compared with canned bean or vegetable soup, which may have 800 milligrams.

CALORIES per serving	360
80% Carbohydrate	50 g
17% Protein	16 g
3% Fat	1 g
CALCIUM	190 mg
IRON	6 mg
SODIUM	188 mg

200 g (7 oz) dried pinto beans
250 g (8 oz) onions, chopped
2 garlic cloves, chopped
4 tablespoons chopped fresh dill
1 bay leaf
¼ teaspoon salt
¼ teaspoon pepper

500 g (1 lb) orange-fleshed sweet
  potatoes, peeled and diced
300 g (10 oz) cabbage, sliced
125 g (4 oz) carrots, sliced
125 g (4 oz) yellow or green
  courgettes, sliced
4 tablespoons chopped parsley

Place the beans in a large pan and add enough cold water to cover them. Cover the pan and leave the beans to soak for 8 hours, or overnight.

Rinse and drain the beans and return them to the pan with enough water to cover them by about 7.5 cm (3 inches). Bring the water to the boil and boil the beans hard for 10 minutes. Rinse and drain the beans, place them in a clean pan and stir in the onions, garlic, 3 tablespoons of the dill, the bay leaf, salt and pepper. Add the sweet potatoes and 2 litres (3½ pints) of water and bring to the boil over medium-high heat. Reduce the heat to medium low, cover the pot and simmer for 35 to 45 minutes, or until the beans are tender.

Add the cabbage, carrots and courgettes and return the soup to the boil. Cook for another 5 to 10 minutes, or until the carrots are tender. Remove and discard the bay leaf, then stir in the parsley. Ladle the soup into four bowls and garnish with the remaining dill.

Makes 4 servings

Cabbage-Carrot-Bean Soup

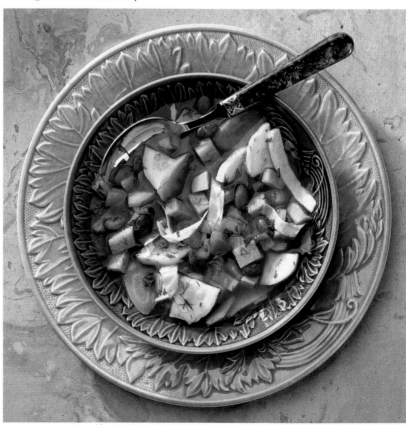

L abels can be a source of confusion when you shop for reduced-calorie foods. "Sugarless" foods may contain glucose or fructose, both sugars. "Light" foods may be light in colour, texture or flavour — but not in calories or fat. "Natural" can mean just about anything. Check the nutrition chart on the packet, then read the ingredients carefully and learn to recognize the hidden sugars, fats and additives you wish to avoid.

GROUND RICE VANILLA PUDDING

If you enjoy ice cream for dessert, try this pudding instead. It has a creamy, rich texture with just a fraction of ice cream's fat and sugar.

30 cl (10 fl oz) skimmed milk
30 g (1 oz) ground rice
60 g (2 oz) sugar
2 teaspoons unsalted butter

½ teaspoon pure vanilla extract
250 g (8 oz) low-fat ricotta cheese
2 kiwi fruits

CALORIES per serving	225
54% Carbohydrate	32 g
18% Protein	10 g
28% Fat	7 g
CALCIUM	253 mg
IRON	1 mg
SODIUM	111 mg

Bring the milk to the boil in a small saucepan over medium heat and slowly stir in the ground rice. Return the milk to the boil, reduce the heat to low and cook, stirring occasionally, for 3 to 4 minutes, or until the mixture is as thick as porridge. Remove the pan from the heat, add the sugar, butter and vanilla and stir until smooth; set aside to cool for about 5 minutes.

Process the ricotta in a food processor or blender until smooth. Add the cooled ground rice and process until smooth. Divide the pudding among four dessert bowls and refrigerate for at least 1 hour.

Just before serving, peel the kiwi fruits and cut them into 5 mm (¼ inch) thick slices. Arrange a few slices on top of each pudding.   Makes 4 servings

Ground Rice Vanilla Pudding

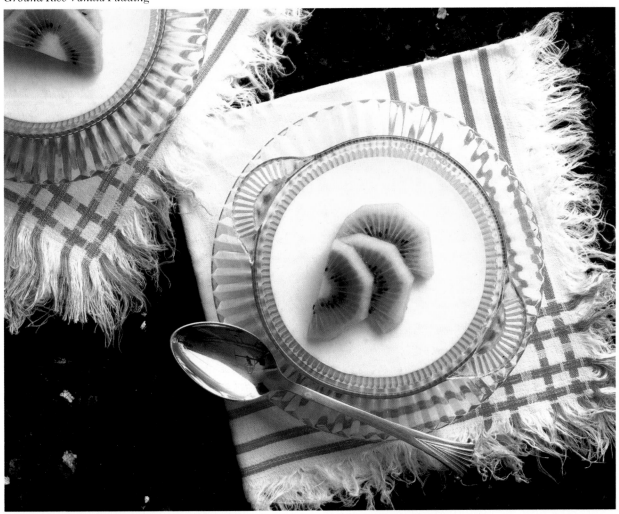

POTATO-VEGETABLE SALAD WITH SALMON ▼

Leaving out the mayonnaise and adding fish and an abundance of low-calorie vegetables turns potato salad into a low-fat dinner dish. Adding salt at the last minute means that you taste it more, so you can use less.

CALORIES per serving	215
54% Carbohydrate	30 g
17% Protein	9 g
29% Fat	7 g
CALCIUM	122 mg
IRON	2 mg
SODIUM	275 mg

12.5 cl (4 fl oz) plain low-fat yogurt

2½ tablespoons olive oil

2 tablespoons finely chopped
   fresh dill

1 tablespoon Dijon mustard

¼ teaspoon pepper

750 g (1½ lb) small red potatoes,
   boiled, peeled and quartered

250 g (8 oz) French beans, cut
   into 2.5 cm (1 inch) lengths and
   blanched

175 g (6 oz) courgettes, grated

125 g (4 oz) carrots, grated

90 g (3 oz) red cabbage, finely
   shredded

90 g (3 oz) radishes, thinly sliced

75 g (2½ oz) frozen broad
   beans, blanched

110 g (3¾ oz) canned salmon

2 shallots, finely chopped

1 tablespoon chopped parsley

¼ teaspoon salt

For the dressing, stir the yogurt, oil, dill, mustard and pepper together in a small bowl until well blended; set aside. Place the potatoes, beans, courgettes, carrots, cabbage, radishes and broad beans in a large bowl and stir to combine. Drain the salmon and add it to the salad. Add the shallots, parsley and dressing and stir gently, breaking up the salmon as little as possible. Add the salt, stir again and serve.

Makes 6 servings

PEAR BREAD PUDDING

When you leave out the butter and use skimmed milk, bread-and-butter pudding is a low-fat, high-carbohydrate dessert. The fibre in the wholemeal bread and pears not only makes you feel full, but also helps lower blood cholesterol levels.

CALORIES per serving	230
70% Carbohydrate	41 g
14% Protein	8 g
16% Fat	4 g
CALCIUM	126 mg
IRON	2 mg
SODIUM	188 mg

2 large eggs

2 tablespoons plain flour

2 tablespoons sugar

25 cl (8 fl oz) skimmed milk

1 teaspoon grated lemon rind

1 teaspoon almond extract

4 slices wholemeal bread,
   preferably slightly stale,
   cut into 1 cm (½ inch) cubes

2 ripe pears (about 550 g/18 oz),
   peeled, cored and cut into
   1 cm (½ inch) cubes

Preheat the oven to 190°C (375°F or Mark 5). Break the eggs into a small bowl and lightly beat them; set aside. For the custard, stir together the flour and sugar in a medium-sized bowl. Gradually add the milk, beating the mixture constantly to prevent lumps from forming. Stir in the eggs, lemon rind and almond extract. Combine the bread cubes and pears and divide them among four 25 cl (8 fl oz) ramekins. Pour the custard over the bread and pears (it will not completely cover them) and stir gently to coat. Bake the puddings for 25 to 30 minutes, or until the custard is set and golden-brown on top. Serve the puddings hot, at room temperature or chilled.

Makes 4 servings

POLENTA WITH CHEESE ▼

A serving of this cheese-topped cornmeal pie provides more than one quarter of the Recommended Daily Amount of calcium for an adult.

CALORIES per serving	190
47% Carbohydrate	24 g
15% Protein	7 g
38% Fat	8 g
CALCIUM	131 mg
IRON	3 mg
SODIUM	204 mg

125 g (4 oz) onion, coarsely chopped
2 garlic cloves, crushed
15 g (½ oz) butter
250 g (8 oz) courgettes, diced
150 g (5 oz) sweet red pepper, diced
¼ teaspoon salt
¼ teaspoon pepper
1 tablespoon chopped fresh dill
2 teaspoons curry powder
100 g (3½ oz) cornmeal
45 g (1½ oz) Cheddar cheese, grated

In a medium-sized, heavy frying pan, sauté the onion and garlic in the butter over medium heat for 4 minutes, or until the garlic is golden. Add the courgettes and red pepper and cook, stirring, for 1 to 2 minutes more, adding up to 2 tablespoons of water, if necessary, to prevent sticking. Add the salt, pepper, dill and curry powder, cover the pan, reduce the heat to low and cook for 5 to 7 minutes, or until the vegetables are tender.

Preheat the grill. Bring 60 cl (1 pint) of water to the boil in a small pan over medium heat. Add the cornmeal, whisking constantly for about 30 seconds to prevent lumps from forming. Continue cooking for 3 to 4 minutes, stirring all the time until the mixture thickens. Pour the cornmeal over the vegetables, stir gently to combine and sprinkle with the cheese. Grill 15 cm (6 inches) from the heat for about 1 minute, or until the cheese is melted.   Makes 4 servings

LENTIL MINESTRONE

Even though this soup contains very small amounts of meat and cheese, it provides 14 grams of protein in a 285-calorie serving. Much of the protein comes from the lentils and macaroni.

CALORIES per serving	285
61% Carbohydrate	44 g
19% Protein	14 g
20% Fat	7 g
CALCIUM	142 mg
IRON	4 mg
SODIUM	563 mg

1 teaspoon olive oil
60 g (2 oz) lean minced beef
250 g (8 oz) onions, coarsely chopped
300 g (10 oz) sweet peppers, coarsely diced
125 g (4 oz) celery, diced
2 garlic cloves, crushed
60 g (2 oz) dried lentils
45 g (1½ oz) white rice
4 small green tomatoes, cut into 2.5 cm (1 inch) cubes
60 g (2 oz) elbow macaroni
1 bay leaf
1 tablespoon lime juice
¾ teaspoon salt
½ teaspoon dried oregano
Black pepper
4 tablespoons grated Parmesan cheese

Heat the oil in a fireproof casserole or heavy-bottomed saucepan over medium heat. Add the beef, onions, sweet peppers, celery and garlic and cook, stirring, for about 5 minutes, or until the vegetables are soft. Stir in the lentils, rice, tomatoes, macaroni, bay leaf and 2 litres (3½ pints) of water, cover the pan and bring to the boil. Reduce the heat and simmer for 45 minutes.

Add the lime juice, salt, oregano, and pepper to taste. Remove and discard the bay leaf, ladle the soup into four bowls and sprinkle with the Parmesan.

Makes 4 servings

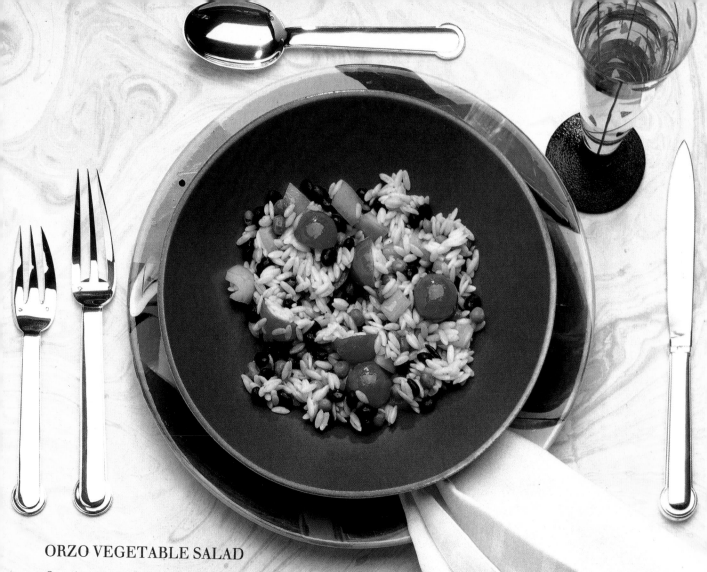

ORZO VEGETABLE SALAD

Orzo is a pasta which is shaped like rice, however, it contains almost double the amount of protein as rice.

300 g (10 oz) orzo
4 tablespoons apple juice
3 tablespoons white wine vinegar
2½ tablespoons vegetable oil
2 teaspoons Dijon mustard
½ teaspoon ground ginger
½ teaspoon pepper
Pinch of salt

250 g (8 oz) cherry tomatoes, halved
175 g (6 oz) cooked black beans (90 g/3 oz dried weight)
150 g (5 oz) cooked peas
1 large sweet yellow pepper, diced

Cook the orzo in a medium-sized saucepan of boiling water for 8 to 10 minutes, or according to the packet directions until *al dente*. Transfer the orzo to a colander, cool under cold running water and set aside to drain.

In a medium-sized bowl, combine the apple juice, vinegar, oil, mustard, ginger, pepper and salt, and stir to combine. Add the tomatoes, beans, peas, yellow pepper and orzo, and stir to combine. Serve the salad either at room temperature or chilled.

Makes 6 servings

CALORIES per serving	325
66% Carbohydrate	55 g
14% Protein	11 g
20% Fat	7 g
CALCIUM	45 mg
IRON	3 mg
SODIUM	81 mg

STUFFED TROUT

Trout is a good source of omega-3 fatty acids, now recognized as useful in helping to reduce blood cholesterol levels.

12.5 cl (4 fl oz) low-sodium
  chicken stock
30 g (1 oz) butter
300 g (10 oz) sweet red peppers,
  diced
150 g (5 oz) mushrooms, sliced
175 g (6 oz) sweetcorn kernels
125 g (4 oz) yellow or green
  courgettes, sliced

100 g (3½ oz) spring onions,
  chopped
2 garlic cloves, chopped
150 g (5 oz) wholemeal bread
  cubes
One 750 g (1½ lb) trout,
  cleaned, rinsed and patted dry
  with paper towels
1 lemon, halved

CALORIES per serving	315
44% Carbohydrate	37 g
29% Protein	24 g
27% Fat	10 g
CALCIUM	85 mg
IRON	4 mg
SODIUM	357 mg

Preheat the oven to 200°C (400°F or Mark 6). Bring the stock to the boil in a large pan over medium-high heat. Add the butter, peppers, mushrooms, sweetcorn, courgettes, spring onions and garlic, and cook, stirring constantly, until the mixture returns to the boil. Remove the pan from the heat and stir in the bread. Transfer three quarters of the stuffing to a large, shallow baking dish and pat it into an even layer. Place the trout on top and fill the cavity of the fish with the remaining stuffing. Cover with foil and bake for 20 to 25 minutes, or until the fish flakes when tested with a fork. Squeeze the juice of one lemon half over the trout; slice the other half for garnish.   Makes 4 servings

Stuffed Trout

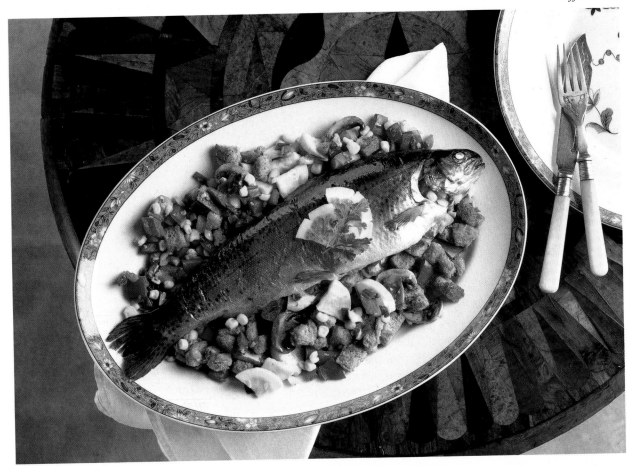

TURKEY SANDWICH WITH CRANBERRY CHUTNEY ▼

Lean turkey breast is one of the lowest-calorie choices for a meat sandwich. The home-made chutney has much less sugar than bottled cranberry sauce, which may have as much as 4 tablespoons of sugar per serving.

1 small apple, washed and cored
1 small seedless orange, washed
45 g (1½ oz) cranberries
2 teaspoons sugar
90 g (3 oz) mushrooms, sliced
8 slices wholemeal bread
1 tablespoon soft margarine

125 g (4 oz) cooked turkey breast,
    thinly sliced
125 g (4 oz) carrots, grated
2 tomatoes, sliced
125 g (4 oz) cos lettuce, torn into
    bite-sized pieces

CALORIES per serving	245
63% Carbohydrate	41 g
23% Protein	15 g
14% Fat	4 g
CALCIUM	95 mg
IRON	3 mg
SODIUM	293 mg

For the chutney, cut the apple and orange into large chunks and place them in a food processor or blender. Add the cranberries and sugar, and process, pulsing the machine on and off, for about 20 seconds, or until the fruits are coarsely chopped and blended; set aside. In a small non-stick frying pan cook the mushrooms with 1 tablespoon of water over medium heat, stirring often, for 3 to 5 minutes, or until softened.

Spread each slice of bread with some of the margarine. Divide the turkey among four of the slices and top with the mushrooms, carrots, tomatoes and lettuce. Spread the remaining slices of bread with the chutney and place them on top of the filling. (If making the sandwiches in advance, do not add the chutney until just before serving, or it will soak through the bread.) Cut the sandwiches in half and serve immediately.   Makes 4 servings

PEACH AND OATMEAL CRISP

Heavy pastry and whipped cream can turn fruit into a high-fat dessert. Try this crisp oatmeal crust and yogurt topping instead. An added dividend: the fibre found in oats has been shown to lower blood cholesterol.

350 g (12 oz) peach slices
4 tablespoons currants
1 tablespoon honey
¼ teaspoon ground cinnamon
¼ teaspoon pure vanilla extract
75 g (2½ oz) rolled oats

3 tablespoons plain flour
1½ teaspoons light brown sugar
4 teaspoons butter or margarine
25 cl (8 fl oz) plain low-fat yogurt
1 teaspoon orange juice

An occasional indulgence in gourmet foods can help you stick to your low-calorie diet by keeping you from feeling deprived. Oysters are an example of such a food with outstanding nutritional benefits: they provide good amounts of iron, copper and zinc, contain cholesterol-lowering fish oil and have only about 10 calories each.

Preheat the oven to 170°C (325°F or Mark 3). Reserving eight thin peach slices for the garnish, combine the remaining peaches, the currants, honey, cinnamon and vanilla in a medium-sized bowl, then spread the mixture evenly in a 20 cm (8 inch) square tin. For the topping, stir together the oats, flour and sugar in a small bowl, then work in the butter with your fingers until the mixture is crumbly. Sprinkle the topping over the peaches and bake for 45 minutes, or until the topping is browned. Let the crisp cool for 5 minutes. Meanwhile, stir together the yogurt and orange juice in a small bowl. Divide the peach crisp among four plates and top each serving with a quarter of the yogurt mixture and two of the reserved peach slices.   Makes 4 servings

CALORIES per serving	275
70% Carbohydrate	49 g
11% Protein	8 g
19% Fat	6 g
CALCIUM	135 mg
IRON	2 mg
SODIUM	86 mg

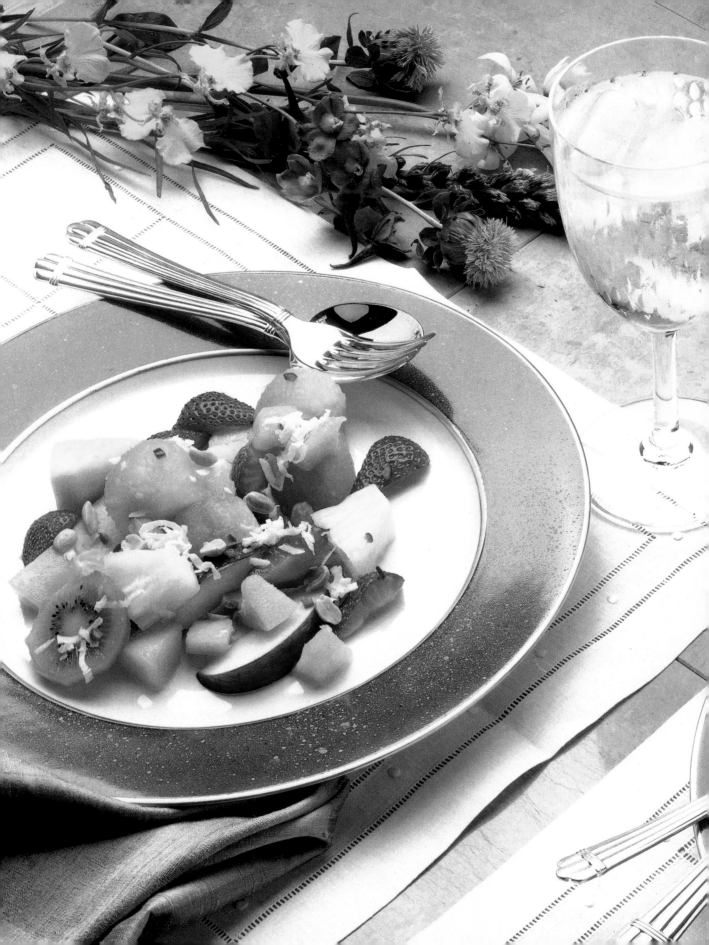

INDONESIAN-STYLE FRUIT SALAD

Even with coconut and peanuts (traditional Indonesian ingredients), this fruit salad still derives only 16 per cent of its calories from fat. It is also an exceptional source of potassium and vitamins A and C.

CALORIES per serving	345
79% Carbohydrate	75 g
5% Protein	5 g
16% Fat	7 g
CALCIUM	81 mg
IRON	2 mg
SODIUM	28 mg

1 small fresh green chili pepper, finely chopped
4 tablespoons freshly squeezed lime juice
3 tablespoons honey
2 Red Delicious apples (about 350 g/12 oz)
1 small honeydew melon
600 g (1¼ lb) fresh strawberries

4 kiwi fruits
2 mangoes
600 g (1¼ lb) fresh pineapple chunks, or drained juice-packed pineapple chunks
45 g (1 ½ oz) shredded fresh or unsweetened desiccated coconut
4 tablespoons roasted peanuts

For the dressing, combine the chili with 3 tablespoons of the lime juice and the honey in a small bowl; set aside. Core but do not peel the apples and cut them into 1 cm (½ inch) cubes. Place them in a small bowl and toss with the remaining lime juice. Cut the honeydew melon into balls or 2.5 cm (1 inch) cubes. Place the melon pieces in a large bowl. Wash, hull and quarter the strawberries and add them to the bowl. Peel the kiwi fruits and mangoes, cut them into bite-sized pieces and add them to the bowl. Add the apples, pineapple and dressing and toss well. Divide the salad among six plates, sprinkle with the coconut and peanuts and serve.

Makes 6 servings

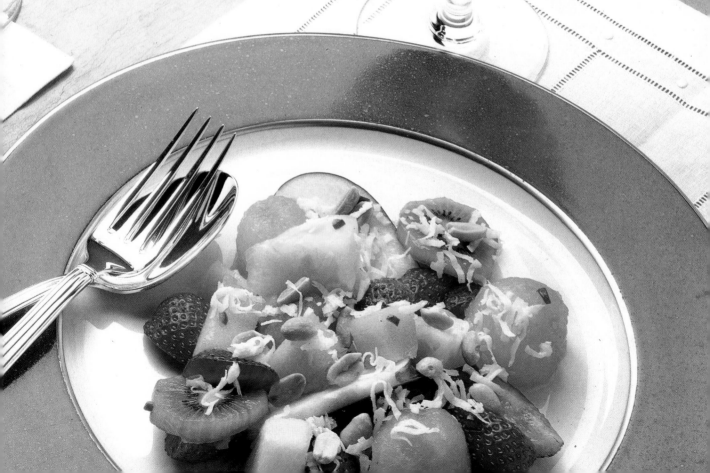

CREAMED SPINACH WITH ONIONS

Serve this vegetable mixture as a side dish, or make it a light meal by doubling the portion and having some wholemeal bread with it.

500 g (1 lb) spinach, washed and trimmed	2 tablespoons plain flour
15 g (½ oz) butter	12.5 cl (4 fl oz) skimmed milk
350 g (12 oz) onions, finely chopped	½ teaspoon grated nutmeg
	¼ teaspoon pepper

Bring 25 cl (8 fl oz) of water to the boil in a medium-sized saucepan over medium-high heat. Add the spinach, and cook, stirring constantly, for 1 to 2 minutes, or until the spinach is wilted. Transfer the spinach to a colander and cool under cold running water. Drain and squeeze the excess water from the spinach. Finely chop the spinach; set aside. Rinse and dry the saucepan. Melt the butter in the pan over medium heat, add the onions, and cook, stirring, for 1 minute. Add the flour and cook, stirring constantly, for 2 minutes. Gradually add the milk and continue to stir for 2 to 3 minutes more, or until the sauce is thick and smooth. Add the spinach, nutmeg and pepper, and cook, stirring, for 2 to 3 minutes, or until the spinach is heated.   Makes 4 servings

CALORIES per serving	95
51% Carbohydrate	13 g
18% Protein	5 g
31% Fat	4 g
CALCIUM	141 mg
IRON	3 mg
SODIUM	112 mg

P*arsley, often used as a garnish, is an underrated source of nutrients. Thirty grams (1 oz) — just 5 calories' worth — fulfils your daily requirement for vitamin C and half your vitamin A requirement. It also supplies good amounts of iron, calcium and potassium. To increase your consumption of fresh parsley, think of it as a vegetable: add plenty of coarsely chopped leaves to green salads, tuna or chicken salad, or stir them into soups and sauces.*

PILAFF WITH MARINATED STEAK

Rump steak is one of the leanest cuts of beef, with less fat than porterhouse or T-bone steak. Although marinating helps tenderize it, rump steak cannot be cooked beyond the medium-rare stage without toughening.

2 teaspoons vegetable oil	25 cl (8 fl oz) low-sodium chicken stock
1 teaspoon lemon juice	
1 teaspoon low-sodium soy sauce	500 g (1 lb) broccoli florets
	8 canned water chestnuts, drained and sliced
1 teaspoon finely chopped fresh ginger root	30 g (1 oz) spring onions, sliced
1 teaspoon crushed garlic	2 teaspoons margarine
150 g (5 oz) lean rump steak	¼ teaspoon salt
250 g (8 oz) white rice	Pepper to taste

In a small non-reactive bowl, stir together the oil, lemon juice, soy sauce, ginger and garlic. Add the steak, cover the bowl and set aside in a cool place to marinate for 1 hour, or refrigerate for at least 2 hours.

About 30 minutes before serving, cook the rice. Bring the stock and 40 cl (14 fl oz) of water to the boil in a medium-sized pan over medium-high heat. Add the rice, cover the pan, reduce the heat and simmer for 20 minutes, or until the rice is tender and the water is all absorbed. Meanwhile, steam the broccoli in a vegetable steamer over boiling water for 5 minutes, or until tender; set aside. When the rice is done, stir in the broccoli, water chestnuts, spring onions, margarine, salt and pepper; cover and keep warm.

Preheat the grill. Grill the steak for 4 minutes on each side, brushing it with the marinade as it cooks. Cut the steak against the grain into 5 mm (¼ inch) thick slices and serve it with the pilaff.   Makes 4 servings

CALORIES per serving	365
68% Carbohydrate	66 g
18% Protein	16 g
14% Fat	6 g
CALCIUM	143 mg
IRON	3 mg
SODIUM	162 mg

SOPA SECA

This Mexican "dry soup" is a combination of pasta, prawns and vegetables. A serving provides 4 milligrams of iron and plenty of vitamin C to aid in the absorption of the iron.

CALORIES per serving		325
69% Carbohydrate		56 g
25% Protein		20 g
6% Fat		2 g
CALCIUM		98 mg
IRON		4 mg
SODIUM		267 mg

25 cl (8 fl oz) low-sodium
   chicken stock
2 garlic cloves, chopped
½ teaspoon dried oregano
¼ teaspoon hot red pepper
   flakes
⅛ teaspoon black pepper
200 g (7 oz) unshelled raw prawns

300 g (10 oz) sweet green
   peppers, diced
350 g (12 oz) onions, chopped
400 g (14 oz) canned plum
   tomatoes, with their liquid
250 g (8 oz) vermicelli, broken
   into 5 cm (2 inch) pieces
3 tablespoons chopped
   fresh coriander

To a large frying pan containing 50 cl (16 fl oz) of water, add the stock, garlic, oregano, pepper flakes and black pepper, and bring to the boil over medium heat. Add the prawns and green peppers and cook for 3 minutes, or until the prawns turn bright pink. Using a slotted spoon, remove the prawns and green peppers; set aside. Add the onions and tomatoes with their liquid to the soup and return to the boil over medium-high heat. Add the vermicelli, and cook, stirring frequently, for 8 to 10 minutes, or until it is tender. Return the prawns and peppers to the pan, stir in the coriander and serve.   Makes 4 servings

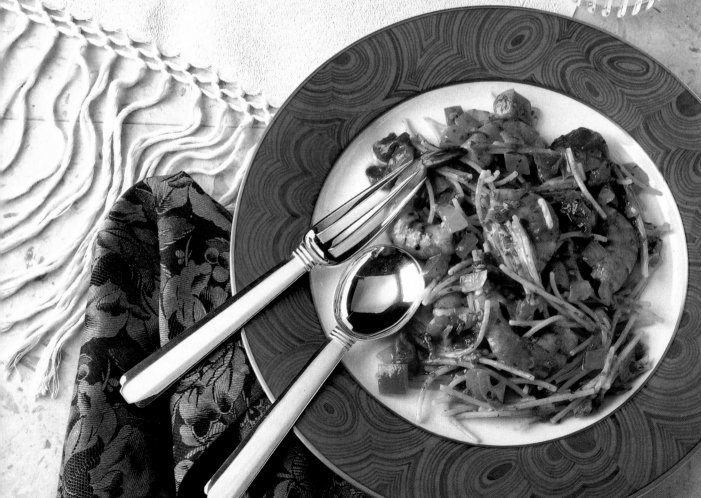

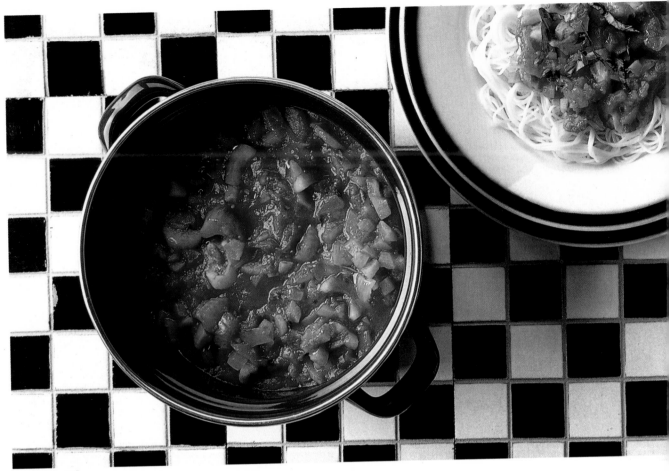

Crab Capellini

CRAB CAPELLINI

Pasta is an excellent calorie-watcher's meal if you keep the sauce low in fat.

CALORIES per serving	370
65% Carbohydrate	61 g
21% Protein	20 g
14% Fat	6 g
CALCIUM	137 mg
IRON	4 mg
SODIUM	481 mg

1 tablespoon olive oil
250 g (8 oz) onions, chopped
2 garlic cloves, chopped
850 g (28 oz) canned plum
  tomatoes
125 g (4 oz) celery, chopped
90 g (3 oz) carrots, chopped

2 tablespoons chopped fresh
  basil
1 bay leaf
250 g (8 oz) dried capellini
  or spaghetti
250 g (8 oz) white crab meat
Black pepper to taste

Heat the oil in a medium-sized saucepan over medium heat. Add the onions and garlic, and sauté for 5 minutes, or until golden. Add the tomatoes and their liquid, the celery, carrots, 1 teaspoon of the basil and the bay leaf, and bring to the boil. Reduce the heat to low and simmer, partially covered, for 30 minutes, or until the flavours are blended and the sauce is thickened.

Fifteen minutes before serving, cook the capellini in a large pan of boiling water for 8 to 10 minutes, or according to the packet directions until *al dente*. Drain the pasta and divide it among four plates. Put quarter of the crab meat on each portion and top it with the sauce. Sprinkle with the pepper and garnish with the remaining basil.

Makes 4 servings

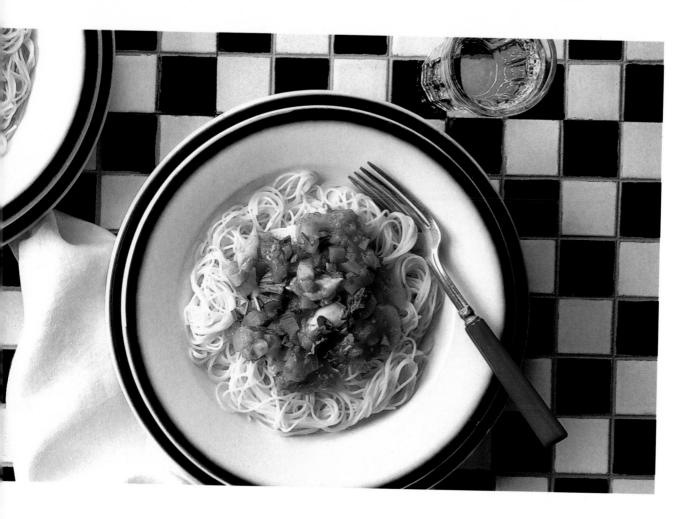

GINGER CHICKEN SOUP ▼

*Prepared without the use of any cooking oil or fat, this soup derives only
10 per cent of its calories from fat.*

1.25 litres (2 pints) low-sodium
  chicken stock
175 g (6 oz) Chinese cabbage,
  shredded
1 large sweet red pepper, cut into
  thin strips
125 g (4 oz) fresh shiitake
  mushrooms, trimmed and sliced
100 g (3½ oz) spring onions,
  thinly sliced

2 tablespoons grated fresh
  ginger root
125 g (4 oz) boneless chicken
  breast, cut into thin strips
175 g (6 oz) soba (Japanese
  buckwheat noodles), cooked
  and drained
350 g (12 oz) watercress leaves,
  chopped
1 tablespoon rice-wine vinegar

CALORIES per serving	255
61% Carbohydrate	37 g
29% Protein	17 g
10% Fat	3 g
CALCIUM	123 mg
IRON	4 mg
SODIUM	102 mg

Bring the stock to a simmer in a large saucepan over medium-high heat. Add
the cabbage, red pepper, mushrooms, spring onions and ginger, and simmer
for 5 minutes. Add the chicken and simmer the soup for 5 minutes more. Stir
in the noodles, watercress and vinegar, and cook for another 2 minutes. Ladle
the soup into four bowls and serve.   Makes 4 servings